*Making the
Moments Count*

Making the Moments Count

Leisure Activities for
Caregiving Relationships

Joanne Ardolf Decker

The Johns Hopkins University Press
Baltimore and London

© 1997 The Johns Hopkins University Press
All rights reserved. Published 1997
Printed in the United States of America on acid-free paper
06 05 04 03 02 01 00 99 98 97   5 4 3 2 1

The Johns Hopkins University Press
2715 North Charles Street
Baltimore, Maryland 21218-4319
The Johns Hopkins Press Ltd., London

Library of Congress Cataloging-in-Publication Data will be found at the end
of this book.
A catalog record for this book is available from the British Library.

ISBN 0-8018-5699-X   ISBN 0-8018-5700-7 (pbk.)

To Mom and Dad, who taught me how to care,
and to Jim, who taught me how to make the moments count

Contents

Acknowledgments

Many people influenced my thinking in quiet ways over the years. Others have been directly involved with this book. I am grateful to all.

Special thanks to Cathy Swoboda, M.S., whose expertise and generous hours of consultation, review, and critique nurtured the kernel of this book into growth and development; Ralph Hall and Bonnie Lund, who believed in this book in its infancy; Carol Jones and Mankato School District 77, who supported my ideas through Project A.L.I.V.E. (Active Leisure in Volunteer Experiences); Pam Determan and V.I.N.E. (Volunteer Interfaith Network Effort) of Mankato, Minnesota, who fed my ideas along the way; Jim Petersen and Kait Klammer, who were helpful and encouraging readers; Jacqueline Wehmueller at the Johns Hopkins University Press, who was my caring, supportive editor.

I am grateful to Dell Bredeson, R.N., who served as a role model early in my career and taught me the importance of meaningful activity in caregiving; S. Lillian Kroll, O.S.F., has been a long-time mentor regarding spiritual activity; Hazel Eggersdorfer and Donna Laue taught me a great deal about ongoing caregiving.

I am deeply grateful to have had meaningful relationships with hundreds of people in my professional work, many of whom became the focus of the cases in these chapters. I continue to be inspired by my students, whose one-to-one volunteer services have shown me the creative possibilities within caregiving roles.

I was fortunate to grow up in a family that made the moments count, and we still do. Special thanks to Mom and Dad for teaching me the importance of caring and for patiently teaching me a wide range of skills; to my sister Miriam and brothers Leo, Gene, and Ed, for nurturing my interests. I am especially grateful for all that we learned about caregiving while caring for Gene. Thank you to his wife Dorothy and daughters Janice and Sandy for letting us share his last weeks of life. My wonderful husband-friend, Jim, is my ongoing support, caregiver, and leisure-time pal. My profound thanks for all your loving contributions to this book and to my life! And thank you, Holy Spirit, for nudging this book into reality.

*Making the
Moments Count*

Making Memories

When my brother Gene was dying from cancer and our family moved into his home to help his wife and daughters care for him, I noticed how precious were the moments when we shared with him a laugh, a poem, snapshots, a memory, a look out the window, a prayer. Those are the moments that last in our memories, now that he is no longer with us.

Esther, a friend and resident at a nearby long-term care facility, always has a pleasant disposition, and she does not seem to mind being alone in her room. I once commented on her contentment, and she replied, "I just love to sit with my memories." Those memories may account for the slight smile she always has on her face.

It seems to me that when all is said and done, it is the memories that come from well-spent moments, large or small, that linger as life's ongoing pleasures. When I conduct workshops I like to ask participants to scan their memories and come up with a "most precious" moment in life. It may have taken place a long time ago or very recently, but it must be considered precious. I give them a minute to find that moment in time and relish it a bit. Then I ask them to raise their hands in response to these questions:

"How many of you were somewhere in nature?" Usually about half raise their hands.

"How many of you were with someone you care for a great deal?" Usually about 90 percent raise their hands.

"How many were at work?" Less than 1 percent ever raise their hands.

"How many would say your precious memory took place in your free time?" Nearly all the hands go up.

I find it interesting that while our society highly values work, when it comes down to life's most precious moments, work is rarely in the picture. Certainly work is a marvelous aspect of life and necessary for livelihood. Our leisure moments, however, give us opportunity to enjoy life, look forward to favorite activities, and develop relationships, interests, and talents—all of which provide more memories for ongoing enjoyment.

Illness, disability, and life difficulties of all kinds complicate leisure time and activity. Yet it is when life is difficult that we are most desperate for joy, laughter, and peace of mind. Caregivers of all ages and in all circumstances know how important they are in providing not only help with feeding, hygiene, and health care, but also in helping to protect and nourish the emotions. This book is designed to help both those needing care and those providing that care by offering simple leisure-time tools to use along the way.

As a therapeutic recreation specialist, I have had opportunity to participate in a growing field called therapeutic recreation service. It is a service that uses education, leisure, and recreation activities to bring about positive changes for better health and more enjoyable living among persons who have illness or disability. Therapeutic recreation specialists (TRSs), sometimes called recreation therapists (RTs), can be found in hospitals, rehabilitation centers, long-term care facilities, mental health centers, prisons, group homes, schools, and community services, and in a wide variety of other human-service settings which help people who, as a result of some limitation, have special needs in the leisure and recreation areas of life. Most therapeutic recreation specialists are certified by the National Council for Therapeutic Recreation Certification. This means that they have been professionally prepared, with a minimum of a bachelor's degree in the field and have passed a certification examination, qualifying them to use the initials *CTRS* after their name.

The therapeutic recreation specialist generally works in a human-service setting with other members of an interdisciplinary team (such as doctors, nurses, social workers, occupational therapists, and physical therapists) to assess people's abilities and interests and set leisure goals that are appropriate for them. The activities that are selected to develop those goals may be done individually or in small group settings and may be done in residential living or after discharge. The goal may be to learn to operate a tape recorder to play favorite music at home or in one's room; to relearn how to care for indoor plants with one good hand following a stroke; or to become very good at using a wheelchair in parks, restaurants, and theaters, for ongoing independence. The TRS helps to modify activities, find suitable adaptive equipment, and teach leisure skills and opportunities for ongoing life satisfaction in spite of illness or disability.

As a therapeutic recreation specialist I have seen firsthand the value of leisure activities in making life's moments count. I recall using art materials and activities to lure Lorraine, a deeply depressed teenager, out of her bed, out of her room, and eventually into counseling; playing Ervin's favorite hymns on the piano each afternoon to entice him from his day-long naps in a corner chair and into a small singing group where eventually he sang solos; hearing Evelyn speak for the first time in a year when a friend brought a small puppy to sit on her lap and lick her hand; watching Violet's face glow with delight while we arranged fresh lilacs in a vase, sniffed deeply the flowers' fragrance, and reminisced about her flower gardens. Such moments bring joy to those involved and make a difference in their lives. Although it is often difficult to prove by means of research data precisely what benefits people gain from such activities, their expressions tell the story of moments that count.

I recall something a co-worker told me early in my career. "Joanne," he said, "you may think you're doing good for the patients here. They get involved in activities and seem to have some fun, but you must realize that when you leave, they'll go back to their old ways. You aren't really doing them any good." Those words rang in my head for days. I was furious! How dare he say I wasn't doing any good! After mulling over that conversation a long time, I concluded that it did not matter whether or not I was making a difference in the long run. I decided my work had to be for the present. I believed then, as I do now, that my work was about helping people be as fully human as possible while we were together. I could not do much to influence what would happen the next day or the next year. But now—in the present moment—I could help them find joy and life satisfaction and give them tools to use in the days ahead, if they had the chance.

As it turned out, the co-worker's gloomy comments served me well over the years. I came to focus on the importance of present moments without paying too much attention to what I could not control thereafter. I don't mean that I whimsically dismissed long-range planning or never thought ahead to what could be gained for the future. Rather, I came to believe in the importance of helping those in my care be as alive as possible in the moments I had with them.

My belief in the importance of each moment has led me to want to share a few leisure tools with others who only have present moments to enjoy. We usually don't know how long we have with those in our care. We can't control what will happen tomorrow, the health changes ahead, mood swings we'll face, or even death. But we are able to make the present moments comfortable, stimulating, alive, and as human as possible. The small moments of shared joy bring relief in the present and build memories to treasure in the future.

Some people think a person who is ill or disabled has so many days, weeks, or months to be endured until death puts an end to the unfortunate circumstance. Some believe it is best to "let him go" rather than painfully maintain connections that will soon be lost; that caregivers should provide good care without emotional attachment. Some think it is useless to engage a person with terminal illness or severe disability in life activities, much less leisure experiences. They may agree with my former co-worker that there is nothing to be gained in the long run and say, "What's the use? She's going to die anyway." Although this approach to caregiving is based on the good intention of "letting go," it is an approach that in many ways brings an end to life well before the heart stops.

Another approach to caregiving is to promote the humanness of the person as long as possible, or as long as the person is able to engage in life experiences, however small. This book supports this more life-affirming approach with an understanding that some who receive care will naturally withdraw not only from leisure but from life's activities in general as a natural step in their departure. Other care recipients, however, are able to participate in activities that support being fully alive and enhance the quality of their lives, even in small moments of "being present" to life. The ideas in this book are tools to use when that is the case.

Whether you are a parent, spouse, child, sibling, cousin, friend, neighbor, home-care worker, or professional caregiver, I encourage you to approach every day "in the present," dedicated to creating good feelings for the person in your care and making memories that will last. Go beyond the general duties required for giving basic care and support quality of life for the person in your care. Look for ways to make each day more interesting for both of you. Then reap the benefits with a smile on your face. Make memories! Make all the moments count!

CHAPTER ONE

Leisure in the Caregiving Process:
What Is It? Who Is It For?
What Does It Do?

Let's consider what leisure is all about and why it is a part of life that should not be neglected, even when a person is ill or disabled. Leisure fits into caregiving in many ways. In this chapter you will find the following:

☆ A discussion of leisure in the caregiving process
☆ An overview of this book
☆ Ideas about how to use the cases in each chapter
☆ A definition of leisure
☆ A discussion of how leisure is important in the caregiving process for the benefit of caregiver and care receiver together as well as each one individually

Anyone who has ever provided the care of someone else knows that leisure is in short supply most of the time, and thus leisure is rarely associated with caregiving. Those who provide care often give up leisure to perform their role, and for most of us that concern is about as far as our thinking goes on the subject of leisure and caregiving. This book looks at leisure differently. It is about *blending* leisure moments *into* the caregiving process. It is about the joy that is available through *shared* leisure experiences.

If, as anthropologist Andrea Sankar has written, caregiving is a relationship in which both parties participate, then shared activities can enhance that relationship through life-affirming, enjoyable activity. The leisure time strategies in this book are designed to connect you, caregiver-to-care receiver, person-to-person, spirit-to-spirit, through smiles, enjoyment, meaning, laughter, and fun.

For most people receiving care, one day is much like another. Their lives are filled with sameness. And much of that sameness involves passive activities that offer little opportunity to take initiative or be active. In 1995 clinical psychologist M. Powell Lawton and associates studied 116 persons who were elderly and disabled and receiving care at home. Family caregivers reported their care recipients' days included rest, TV, radio, and receiving assistance from the caregiver. That's not much to look forward to every day! The study goes on to encourage in-home workers and family caregivers to provide varied activities, social opportunities, and a more stimulating environment. This book will help you do that.

The leisure-time tips offered in the chapters ahead are meant for those moments when the dressing has been accomplished, maintenance activities are finished, the meals are over, and the question comes up: "Now what?" Rather than merely turning on the TV or hoping someone will stop by, you can take an active approach to leisure time to rejuvenate spirits, enjoy interests, build relationships, make memories, and make even life's difficult moments more bearable for everyone involved.

Simple leisure activities can help lighten daily living even in the midst of illness and disability. You may associate leisure with time-consuming, costly activities such as travel, sporting events, and professional entertainment, or you may believe that high levels of mental and physical fitness are necessary for participation. But this book tells a different story. It's about doing everyday things that bring good feelings to all people, whether they are healthy or not, active or not. It's about turning common activities that are sometimes overlooked into favorite activities that satisfy people's needs in everyday life, and you can enjoy leisure moments without needing elaborate equipment and supplies or spending a great deal of time and money. The activities described in this book can be done in most households and can easily be blended into daily living.

This book is addressed to the full range of caregivers: caregiving family members, relatives, friends, neighbors, volunteers, in-home workers, and professional caregivers. It can be useful whether you provide care full time, part time, or occasionally. The role of caregiver varies greatly from one situation to another, yet all caregivers know the feeling of carrying responsibilities. This book is meant to ease the burden, not increase it. The ideas it offers for what to do with short moments available in the course of every day can lighten the burden rather than add more duties to perform. Even in the process of actively providing care there are many opportunities to escape obligations and share life's pleasures with the person in your care. Activities such as watching the sunset, arranging flowers in a vase, eating a picnic in the backyard, planting seeds and watching them grow, solving a mind teaser, or reminiscing over old photos offer lasting moments of simple pleasure. Psychologists Lawton and associates encouraged caregivers to attend to the quality of life of those in their care, because that is what they are there to do. Replacing time that drags with time filled with interesting activities will help caregivers feel better too.

What's Ahead: An Overview of This Book

In the rest of this chapter, after explaining how to use the stories in each chapter, I will spend some time considering the meaning of leisure, an aspect of life that is often neglected and misunderstood. Then I'll turn to a closer look at how leisure affects both the person receiving care and the caregiver.

In Chapter 2, I'll describe a system I developed called the P.I.E.S.S. of Activities, (pronounced like "pies"), composed of the Physical, Intellectual, Emotional, Social, and Spiritual benefits that can be expected when people participate in leisure activities. Chapter 2 also offers the Checklist of Leisure Favorites to help you identify leisure interests— your own as well as those of the person you're caring for. You can use the list to discuss favorite activities enjoyed in the past, and find out which physical, intellectual, emotional, social, and spiritual activities are still desirable and possible. It can give you clues for planning meaningful leisure moments.

The middle chapters are organized according to the P.I.E.S.S. Chapter 3 addresses physical activities and simple ideas for including general body movement into daily living. Chapter 4 highlights intellectual activities including reminiscence and sensory stimulation. Chapter 5 is about using emotional and self-expressive activities to bring out the unique self through activities. Included are suggestions for using humor and building self-esteem. Chapter 6 focuses on social activity and how to include other people, plants, and pets in the social life of your care recipient. Celebrations and activities centered around special events, holidays, and outings can help people with illness or disability stay in touch with family, friends, and the wider community. Chapter 7 discusses spiritual activities and offers many suggestions for uplifting the spirit.

Chapter 8 will help you plan a leisure goal for every day so you and the person in your care both have something to look forward to, and then something to remember fondly. It may be something as simple as carefully roasting marshmallows until golden brown over the burner of your stove or watching birds feed outside the window, but looking forward is key to *living* every day rather than just making it through the day.

In Chapter 9, I will address leisure just for the caregiver, and how support groups can offer information and assistance. There is also discussion about how to ask for help and how to find contact people who can help you find leisure opportunities in your community. My last comments are a few words about the importance of leisure for everyone.

Using the Cases in Each Chapter

As you read along, you will find cases in each chapter that introduce you to both caregivers and people receiving care. The stories are examples of real life situations that illustrate how leisure activities have enhanced other people's lives. Use the cases to "try out" activities that you think might work for you by seeing how they worked out for other people—such as Sarah, whose situation is described below.

In the case of Sarah, you will see how her family and friends found ways to modify her quilt-making activity and keep her interested in her hobby. Although your care receiver's interests or disability may be different from Sarah's, you can apply the information about modifying activities to the person's needs. The specific situations in most of the cases you find in this book will be different from your own, but there is information in every story that applies to your situation. For instance, the case may be about someone who has visual impairment, whereas the person in your care has dementia; your care recipient may be young and struggling with cancer, whereas some stories you come upon will be about older people with a variety of conditions other than cancer. Rather than looking for stories with situations exactly like your own, read the chapters in relation to the physical, intellectual, emotional, social, and spiritual aspects of leisure activities and creatively consider how you can apply the information.

All the stories are written to have applications to *people* and their leisure needs, not specifically to their illnesses or disabilities. In this book activities are not designated as being just for people who have dementia, or just for those who have cancer, or to be done only by people who have had strokes. Leisure activities are for *people* to enjoy according to their unique interests and abilities. The key is to find activities that suit the person, whether it is you or the person in your care. This is not a recipe book, and it will not tell you what to do with every free moment. Instead, it is a book filled with tools for you to apply and enjoy as you daily solve the leisure-time challenges of caregiving for yourself, for your care receiver, and for your relationship to each other.

Making Modifications

Sarah

After a slight stroke, Sarah, who has been a champion quilt maker, currently has no interest whatsoever in sewing or making fiber crafts. Although such activities brought her a great deal of joy earlier in life, now her eyesight and coordination have diminished to the point that she simply is frustrated with those activities. Family members and home health aides have encouraged her, saying her work is still good; but she knows that her product is below her standards. She doesn't want anything substandard with her name on it. Such activities now are just reminders of precious skills lost. Sarah does enjoy the times when family members visit and look at her quilts and crafts, though. Her quilts often bring on stories that are reminiscent of the times when her children wore the dresses and shirts Sarah sewed for them—the pieces of which now make up the quilt designs. Sarah also enjoys looking at the photos of her champion work with friends, family, and aides. The aide who comes on Monday afternoons and helps Sarah change her bedding always takes time to admire Sarah's favorite quilt, which they carefully arrange on top as the bedspread. One of Sarah's granddaughters is in the process of making a quilt and has asked her grandmother for advice from time to time. Sarah seems to enjoy her role as "quilt consultant."

Sometimes an earlier leisure pursuit is best replaced with *related* activity rather than continued as it was. Sarah still has interest in quilts, but no longer wants to make them. Her family, friends, and home health aides help her maintain her interest by engaging her in *related* activities—sharing her art with others who admire it, looking at photos, reminiscing, and giving advice. In the case of your care receiver, it may be necessary to modify some activities in light of current illness or disability. Think of all sorts of activities related to the original interest. For instance, a person who had an interest in fishing may not be able to go out fishing now, but he or she may enjoy looking through outdoor and wildlife magazines, watching videos about fishing, visiting a fishery, reminiscing through photos of "the big ones," telling stories about "the ones that got away," or giving directions to a favorite fishing spot. It is often necessary to simplify activities.

Although your care receiver has an illness or disability, he or she still may be able to do a small portion of an activity. Seek out remaining skills. Find creative ways for the person to share skills and interests. How about making an audio- or videotape telling or showing how to do something—making a pattern for a quilt block, tying flies for trout fishing, or making a favorite spaghetti sauce. Can the person still teach the activity to you or someone else—neighbors, grandchildren, a volunteer? Capitalize on the person's talents so he or she can become an "expert" advisor on the subject. (Chapter 5 has more ideas on this topic).

Plan activities that use the person's remaining abilities. Avoid saying, "Well, she can't get out of the house any more, so she can't go places." Rather, consider the remaining skills, such as, "She can still get around in her own house." Or, "She can still hold a pen or brush to write or paint." Or, "She can still sit by the window to watch people walking by." Denial sometimes comes into play when someone is ill or disabled, and it may be that the caregiver or the person receiving care will have a hard time facing the fact that the person can't do everything that she or he used to do. To avoid frustration—both for you and for the other person—you'll need to choose activities that can be done successfully under the present circumstances. It may take some trial and error to find which activities are possible as well as comfortable and interesting. Don't lose heart if you try something that doesn't work the first time. Next time, you can make adjustments in the activity so you *both* will have more fun.

The Meaning of Leisure

Leisure is a complex term that means different things to different people. If you ask your family or friends how they define *leisure* you will hear some of these responses: doing whatever you want; free time; having fun; relaxing; doing nothing. In his book *Leisure in Your Life: An Exploration*, Geoffrey Godbey emphasizes that the terms *leisure*, *recreation*, and *play* frequently are used interchangeably, further complicating how we understand and discuss leisure. Another leisure educator, John Kelly, in his book *Leisure*, notes three commonly accepted definitions: (1) leisure is understood as discretionary, *free time*; (2) leisure is freely chosen, self-satisfying *activity*; (3) leisure is an *inner experience* of freedom and self-satisfaction. Each one of these definitions carries only part of the meaning, yet self-satisfaction and freedom are essential ingredients of leisure.

For the sake of clarity in this book, I have chosen to use the terms *leisure* and *leisure time* to mean "freedom from necessity." *Leisure time*, here, will refer to those blocks of time, however large or small, when there is no "have to" involved, and you have choices about what to do and how to do it, when you have freedom to pursue what is satisfying to you. *Leisure activity* will refer to freely chosen, enjoyable activity that is free from necessity. When I use the term *leisure experience*, I mean the inner experience of good feelings that results from leisure activities; feelings such as joy, refreshment, freedom, control, competence, and wholeness. Perhaps you have other names for the good feelings you associate with leisure. They are just as valid as the good feelings I named above.

What we do as leisure activity varies greatly from one person to another. Some of us engage in traditional leisure pursuits such as sports, games, and outings and find them satisfying. Others enjoy certain activities that would make some people question our sanity. In his free time my husband cuts wood and splits it with a sledge hammer and wedge. Friends wonder why he does such hard work the old-fashioned way. But for him it is not work at all; rather, it is free from necessity. He does it purely for fitness and enjoyment, not because we have to have the wood to stay warm. There is no "have to" involved.

We cannot tell whether or not someone's activity is producing a leisure outcome for the participant merely by observing it. As you pass a tennis court, you do not know who is having a wonderful time, who is actually working by trying to improve every move, or who is dreading the game but going through the motions anyway. Outer appearance does not tell the leisure story. Rather, the person's attitude toward and the inner sense surrounding the activity determine whether or not it is leisure.

How we think about what we do makes the difference. Our attitude determines whether or not an activity is truly leisure. This being the case, it follows that, because we can find enjoyment regardless of the specific activities, our list of leisure activities can be endless. In other words, our range of leisure activities is broader than the traditional recreational pursuits often understood as leisure. They are not the only way we can get the good feelings we associate with leisure.

In 1985 therapeutic recreation educators Carol Peterson and Scout Lee Gunn described a variety of actions which, depending on our attitude at the time, may become "nontraditional leisure experiences." Most of us enjoy these activities on a regular basis:

⇨ socializing, visiting
⇨ preparing food, eating, entertaining
⇨ shopping
⇨ caring for living things: plants, pets and others
⇨ self-care activities such as bathing, dressing, primping
⇨ home improvement and maintenance such as rearranging furniture, cleaning, gardening
⇨ self-improvement activity: reading, learning, going to workshops
⇨ relaxing, appreciating, praying, meditating
⇨ leadership and community service

⇨ intimacy
⇨ fantasizing
⇨ doing nothing

In fact, most of us engage in these nontraditional leisure-time activities far more often than we pursue traditional recreation. For example, I enjoy playing volleyball, but when I play I must gather a group and schedule a time in a certain place. As a result, I rarely play volleyball. On a daily basis, though, I can make many moments into leisure experiences. If I have enough time, I can take a long hot shower in the morning, enjoy my cup of coffee while I dress, comb my hair this way and that while making faces in the mirror, converse with my husband over breakfast, fuss with my plants, and stroll through my garden in the summertime. These are the moments I find rejuvenating, but only when I have a leisurely frame of mind. If I wake up late and make myself rush through my morning tasks, they are not leisure but rather turn into chores to be accomplished. They have "necessity" rather than "leisure" written all over them.

I remember one of my students' surprise when she learned the meaning of nontraditional leisure activities. She was amazed that leisure was more available to her than she thought. We can feel deprived of leisure experience if we think it means participating only in such things as traveling, eating out, playing sports, or going to parties, the movies, concerts, or ball games. Although such activities can be very satisfying (and I highly encourage them), they are usually not as available to us as are the nontraditional activities built into every day. Nontraditional leisure activities are very much available in the home and in small group settings, where caregiving often takes place.

The Importance of Leisure

For Caregiver and Care Receiver Together

Most often the shared activities of caregiver and the person receiving care are not leisure activities but rather maintenance and tasks of daily living. Most research on the activities of caregiving has focused on two issues: the chores caregivers perform and the stress they experience. Very little research has explored the more human experience of caregivers and the meaning they attach to their activities. The intimacy of the caregiving relationship lends itself to sharing common experiences which can turn into enjoyable moments. Leisure can connect people because they are doing something together. The relationship is a key element of caregiving.

In his book *Leisure Wellness*, C. Forrest McDowell explained a relationship in terms of a mathematical formula: $1 + 1 = 3$ (me + you = us). McDowell shows that in this view of a relationship each person has an individual identity as well as a special joint relationship with the other person. If we relate that formula to caregiving, the caregiver is one party (me), the care receiver is the second party (you), and their joint relationship forms a third entity (us). That third entity consists of the unique experiences we share together, unknown to others. It is the goal of all relationships to have positive experiences, one after another, to build a strong "us" as the third entity. That is what we intend to do when we invite a friend to lunch, go for a walk with a child, or play a table game with a family member. We anticipate the activity will help strengthen our relationship with the other while we share a good time.

The services that caregivers provide are tightly packaged in intense personal relationships. The person-to-person connection is an area of caregiving research that is receiving more attention from researchers who suggest that caregiving often *creates* rather than results from a close personal relationship. Human development and aging specialist Leonard I. Pearlin and his associates at the University of California, San Francisco, explained in 1990 that giving care to someone is an extension of caring about that person, and that caring and caregiving are present in all relationships where people attempt to protect or improve each other's well-being. If you think about it, it makes sense to use opportunities in the caregiving process to build close relationships.

In certain situations, the mental or emotional condition of the person receiving care makes it difficult for there to be a real two-way relationship. However, doing things together can build a nonverbal bridge to connect those involved through familiar experience. Don't underestimate the positive feelings that come from shared experiences such as playing catch with a softball, singing together while preparing a snack, watching squirrels play in trees outside the window, eating ice cream cones together, identifying relatives in old photos, or winding a music box and listening together to the delicate sounds.

Sometimes, when we do pleasant things together, we find common ground beyond illness or disability. Sherry L. Dupuis and Alison Pedlar are family and leisure researchers who did a study in 1995 asking family members to join in a regular singing and reminiscence activity with their institutionalized relatives who had Alzheimer's Disease. They found that (a) family members reported their visits went better; (b) the music program helped them cope with the family member's condition; and (c) they felt closer to their family member because of what they experienced while singing together and reminiscing about the songs. This study points again to the important "connecting" function of leisure activity. Doing things together can connect you, caregiver-to-care receiver, through shared experiences that produce joy and build the "us" of the relationship.

In an article he called "Songs of Innocence and Experience" which appeared in the March 26, 1996, edition of the *Wall Street Journal*, John Carter described a bonding experience he shared with his mother. A shortened version of his article was printed in the August 1996 edition of the *Reader's Digest*, with the title "Singing with Mom." I have included it here because it illustrates very well the connecting power of shared leisure experience—in this case, singing.

Singing with Mom

Mom's memory went wild after my dad died. Later on, she no longer knew me, her only living child. And yet she was always delighted to see me, and believed me completely when I said, "It's your son, John, Mom."

My 87-year-old mother's recollections of an extraordinarily vibrant life were increasingly elusive. She told me a wonderful story about a cruise she and her sister, both schoolteachers, took around Cape Horn in 1925:

"We were able to save money on our small salaries because we lived very simply at home with our mother. On the ship we'd walk on the deck in the morning, play badminton in the afternoon and then stay up late because the nights were warm and clear and there was moonlight—and starlight. I met a lovely young man, and we had a very sweet romance, standing at the railing in the evening, singing songs together."

This was a real memory, dormant for many years. But soon Mom began to talk of an imaginary second husband. She and my father had been married only briefly, she said—though actually she and Dad were married for 50 years.

She was shocked each time I reminded her that I lived in California. She was delighted by every bit of family news I gave her—and delighted all over again if I repeated the same news a moment later. Beyond that she had almost nothing to say.

Visits became painful. I wanted to spark her memory with vivid images—"I know you remember the Christmasberry tree in the back yard . . . ." I wanted her to remember, too, new stories about my kids and my life in the West.

She remembered none of it, sensed that she was failing me and became agitated. Sometimes visits lasted only 20 minutes: I ran through all my special news, told her I loved her, and didn't know what else to say.

A few years ago, out of desperation, I began to sing to her, quietly, shyly. I brought along the copy of the old *Fireside Book of Folk Songs* that used to perch on Mom's baby grand piano in the 1950's.

Sitting up straight, I sang "Loch Lomond" to my mother that day, filling my lungs, enunciating, remembering her at the piano, feeling the music glow within me.

To my astonishment Mom began to sing along, reading the words above my finger, then singing from memory.

Mom was ecstatic as we sang, and so was I. She'd clap her hands as we finished a song, and once took my hands in hers, looked into my eyes and said, "I never knew there could be such sweetness in a human relationship."

Another time, as we rested between songs, I said '90's style, "This is kinda nice." She drew herself upright, indignant at my sloppy language. "*Kinda* nice? This is more than *kinda* nice!"

During visits after that, we did nothing but make music. On my wooden recorder I conjured up more than a hundred of the songs she had originally taught me—"Red River Valley," "The Band Played On," "I'll Take You Home Again, Kathleen"—songs Mom had learned as many as 80 years ago.

Her voice floated with my recorder's melody, two frail sopranos at play. She sang without words, her voice itself an instrument.

Once, near the top of "Danny Boy," her clear voice sailed way above my high note, but exactly right, a wild perfect harmony she broke by sailing, for a timeless instant, even higher. She stopped as though she had screamed.

Shocked at herself, she looked at me to see if what she had done was okay. Yes, I said with my eyes, as I wound down through the last chorus of "Danny Boy." Mom looked back with eyes full of wonder, as she must have looked at me on the first day of my life.*

For the Care Receiver Individually

Just because someone is ill or disabled does not mean the need for leisure disappears. A person remains a person no matter what, and people of all ages and health conditions need a chance to enjoy life and stimulating activity to the extent they are able. Although illness and disability complicate leisure time and activities, stimulation is key to feeling alive, whether it is physical, intellectual, emotional, social, or spiritual stimulation. "Quality of life" is a difficult concept to define because the definition depends on the point of view of the individual. In an admirable effort to define quality of life, however, activity consultant Letitia T. Jackson in 1991 identified several elements of life that are commonly associated with quality of life and are also related to leisure. They are: relationships, community involvement, intellectual development, self-expression, socializing, and meaningful activity. Without quality-of-life opportunities, life with illness or disability becomes just a series of grim tasks to be repeated day after day. In 1985 Sefra Kobrin Pitzele wrote about her own experiences in learning to live with chronic illness and made this point by transforming the old saying "All work and no play makes Jack a dull boy" into "All seriousness and no fun makes an ill person boring"—and, I might add, *bored.*

A day filled only with rest, TV, and waiting for care lacks the stimulation many people find necessary to provide motivation to face the day. But if lunch on the porch with a friend is planned into the day, there is something to look forward to, and good reason to get out of bed, dress for the visit, and make it to the porch and back again. It is moments like this that "count" because of looking forward to something, enjoying the actual activity, and then fondly remembering the special event. Such a day will go by more quickly and will mean more than a day spent resting or dwelling on pain.

In their study of elderly care receivers' daily activities, Lawton and associates found that only 3 of 116 had any recreation on the day of the survey. Only passive activities (rest, TV, radio, receiving care) consumed their day. This is a grim picture of the life of those receiving care, and especially difficult to contemplate if it reflects what life is like in *most* caregiving situations. This study not only points out a sad situation but shows the need for more variety in the lives of those receiving care.

Leisure activities can not only help to divert attention away from sameness, pain, and difficulties, but there are many other benefits to be derived from participating in activities. Catherine P. Coyle and fellow researchers in 1991 summarized numerous studies of therapeutic recreation programs which point to benefits for participants. Those participating in these programs experienced improvements in physical health, cognitive functioning, psychosocial health, personal and life satisfaction, and benefits related to society and health care systems. The value of participating in activities will be documented more clearly in the following chapters as we discuss various activity ideas.

Perhaps the most basic reason, though, to engage your care receiver in leisure activities is simply to help him or her feel better. "Feeling better" is an experience that does not easily lend itself to research, and it may be interpreted in many ways. Often, when we say we feel better, we mean that we are experiencing some improvement in physical functioning, that we have less pain than we had, or that we've enjoyed an emotional lift. Sometimes it is a combination of these things that leaves a person with the sensation of feeling better. Sickness, pain, supervision, loss of freedom, and emotional "lows" are often part of a care receiver's life; and, as the caregiver, you do what you can to help him or her feel better. Providing good care for body, mind, and soul is your way of doing that. You are in a position to influence the person's experience of feeling better, in more ways than one. A powerful way to impact how a person feels is to try to build self-esteem—the person's sense of self-worth. Most of us would agree that when we do what we want to do, we feel good about ourselves. It's that way for your care receiver, too. When you include even simple leisure activities in caregiving, you will be helping the person feel good about himself or herself.

Be more concerned about how the person feels while doing the activity than about the exact way to do it. There seldom is only one way to do an activity or only one perfect activity to do with a person. Rather, keep in mind that still being able to do things and enjoy moments of small pleasure will help to maintain the person's humanness and dignity. I believe building self-esteem is the "bottom line"—the most basic purpose—behind all the leisure experiences you share with the person in your care. It is an important way to help that person feel better.

For the Caregiver Individually

By now I hope it's clear how important leisure is as a component of life, but leisure easily is neglected in the caregiving process. In fact, we often overlook our leisure needs even during more ordinary times because life's many demands require leaving something out. Leaving out time for enjoyment may be easier to do than leaving out something else. We convince ourselves there is nothing to be lost by filling every waking hour with tasks to be accomplished. Yet, taking time to refresh oneself makes life worth living. The leisure activities you share with the person in your care can be just as important to you as to the other person. You, too, need a change of pace once in a while and a break from the sameness of your routines.

I am reminded of the story of a man who found his friend cutting down trees in the woods. He was having a difficult time of it because his saw was very dull. "Why don't you stop a while and sharpen your saw?" the man asked his friend. "I can't do that," he said. "There's so much wood to cut here; I don't have time to stop and sharpen my saw!" In this situation, most of us would tell the friend he is being foolish. Allowing leisure into your life is like sharpening that saw. It provides opportunity to leave concerns behind, sharpen your wits, enjoy smiles, fun, and laughter, and put *balance* into your life. Like the teeter-totter that is off balance, with too much weight on one side, caregiving can pull you down, requiring an up-hill climb in order to keep going. But if you can balance out the one-sidedness of that weight, you will cope better and be able to keep going.

A great deal has been written about caregiver burden, the impact of stress on caregivers' leisure time, and the importance of caregivers' taking care of themselves so they can better care for others. Although this is an important topic, I have chosen to address it in the final chapter, since this book is primarily about the *joint* leisure experiences of caregivers and their care receivers. In Chapter 9, I will discuss not only the importance of leisure for caregivers, independent from their care receivers, but the importance of leisure information and activities in support groups for caregivers.

When you plan some leisure activities into your caregiving days, you will do that because you know how those activities can help the person in your care. But it is equally important that you see how valuable those leisure moments are for *you*, too. Adding some variety to the other person's days will help you feel you are doing something worthwhile. You can have things to look forward to, and sharing a little fun together will break the routine for both of you. It will give you a chance to feel better about each other, and when you feel good about the person in your care, you can go about your tasks with a lighter, more loving heart. When you do familiar activities together, you can feel things are more normal, perhaps more like they used to be. You will be making memories that will last for years to come. You can make the moments count, not only for the person in your care, but for yourself too.

Summary

Leisure, loosely defined as freedom from necessity, does not have to be neglected in the caregiving process. Small moments of enjoyment *can* be created, and they benefit caregivers and those receiving care by helping them bond and providing mutual satisfaction. There are far more potentially enjoyable activities than the traditional recreational activities that automatically come to mind and that are usually associated with leisure. With an open frame of mind and a leisurely attitude, a variety of daily activities can be turned into nontraditional leisure experiences to help build relationships and decrease the burden of tasks at hand.

Leisure can bring benefits to the relationship between caregiver and care receiver by connecting them in shared experiences. Leisure opportunities can divert a care receiver's attention from pain or boredom and provide something to look forward to. Leisure moments give caregivers time to rejuvenate and "recharge their batteries" so their work is more effective and less stressful.

CHAPTER TWO

Assessing Leisure Favorites

Chapter 1 explored the meaning of leisure and how important leisure is in the caregiving process. Now it's time to think about how to make leisure "come alive" in your own caregiving situation. So, in Chapter 2 you will find the following:

☆ Explanation of the P.I.E.S.S. System of activities—the physical, intellectual, emotional, social, and spiritual benefits expected from participating in leisure activities

☆ Directions for being an "investigator of fun" for the person in your care

☆ The Checklist of Leisure Favorites, to help you gather information about leisure patterns and interests

"What do you like to do for fun?" is a question we frequently ask when we want to learn more about someone, what motivates them, what gets them up and out and doing things, what puts a smile on their face. In the caregiving process, this is an important question to ask both yourself and your care receiver. The answer to this question will help you decide how to set up situations for enjoyment. There are many, many possibilities, once you find out what someone likes to do. When you think about doing something for fun, consider what benefits can result from doing the activity. Not only can activities be enjoyable, they can help us meet a variety of our human needs.

Knowing the Whole Person

As human beings, we are complex, and have a wide variety of needs and modes of expression. Those who study human behavior have grouped our actions into three main categories called "the behavioral domains." In textbooks, the behavioral domains are usually sorted into the *psychomotor* (physical), *cognitive* (intellectual/mental), and *affective* (social and emotional) domains, as supported by the therapeutic recreation educators Richard Kraus and John Shank in 1992, and Carol Peterson and Scout Lee Gun in 1983. I first learned about behavioral domains when I was a young student preparing to be a teacher. I was taught that the behavioral domains could help me to "take apart" a person and see the "pieces" and then know whether or not I was reaching the "whole person"—meaning every aspect of the human being. The behavioral domains could help me target learning experiences toward particular outcomes and guide students' learning toward specific goals. This was preferable to randomly doing things and hoping students would learn from the activities. As it turned out, I made it a habit to think about which "part" of the student each activity could develop. That made it possible for me to try to reach the whole person.

Let me illustrate these concepts with a few examples. When I taught reading, I used reading methods to help students *cognitively* recognize letters, combine sounds, interpret meanings, understand and retain information. At the same time, in order to ensure interest in reading, I selected material that appealed to students' emotional levels, and I tried to make the experience meaningful and fun so as to meet their *affective* needs in a variety of ways. For example, depending upon the story, I would sometimes stop for a moment of quiet appreciation of something in the story that put the students in touch with their own inner spirits. Or, after reading a story, sometimes I asked students to act out a scene in a small group to develop self-expression and social skills. Getting up and away from their desks also gave them a little physical movement as a *psychomotor* change of pace. By paying attention to each behavioral domain, it was possible to reach the whole person, even through an activity such as reading, which at first glance seems to be only an intellectual activity.

Later in my career, when I became a therapeutic recreation specialist, I continued to use the behavioral domains. People I worked with in treatment or in residential settings had limitations that interfered with their ability to enjoy leisure in life. By recognizing the nature of their limitations (physical, intellectual, social, or emotional) I could select activities that helped, in very focused ways, to diminish their problems in specific areas while simultaneously improving the whole self. I was better able to choose useful, active games to improve a coordination problem; help someone without speech to express himself or herself through music, art, or poetry; or set up occasions that would help someone gain confidence in social situations.

Leisure can provide a framework for becoming engaged in life. For example, when Beverly, a newly arrived group home resident, isolated herself in her room saying, "I don't know anyone here," it wasn't difficult to see that she had a social need—to get acquainted with those around her. To help with this need, I took other people to her room, one at a time for brief visits, so Beverly could get to know them. At the same time, I also continued to invite her to join us for walks, and after a few days she knew a few people by name and seemed to feel comfortable enough to accompany a small group on a walk. After that, she not only came out of her room, but joined others for meals, activities, and conversation. Because I understood that Beverly had a social need, I could concentrate on a specific social strategy to meet that need. I also tried, by means of the frequent visits to her room and invitations for walks, to increase her trust in me—which touched the emotional side of Beverly. Then, when she trusted both me and others enough to come out of her room, she was able to be more active socially as well as physically. Because we cannot *really* take a person apart and work with just one of the domains at a time, it is often the case that a change in one area brings a change in another, as we see in Beverly's case. Still, being able to target what is needed according to the domains makes it possible to help someone with a specific need. That is how knowing about the behavioral domains can be useful.

When I began to teach college students majoring in therapeutic recreation, I realized how important it was for them to understand and use the behavioral domains, just as I had over the years. But the terms *psychomotor, cognitive,* and *affective* always seemed overly technical and abstract to me and to students. So, to help students understand the behavioral domains in a more useful way, I developed the P.I.E.S.S. System, which covers the traditional behavioral domains less technically and in greater detail. "P.I.E.S.S." is an acronym for the behavioral domains. Although it has an extra "s," I pronounce it "pies," because it carries the idea of pieces that fit together into a whole, which in this case is not a pie but a human being. Also, using the term "pies" adds a little fun to the term and makes it easy to understand, remember, and use. This is how my system compares to the traditional view of the behavioral domains:

Traditional Behavioral Domains	*The P.I.E.S.S. System*
Psychomotor	Physical
Cognitive	Intellectual
	$\Bigl\{$ Emotional/Expressive
Affective	Social
	Spiritual

If you include activities from all the P.I.E.S.S. into leisure moments in caregiving, both you and the person you care for will enjoy a variety of experiences. At the same time, you can develop interests and skills that serve the whole person—all of the categories of our human behavior. The chapters ahead will help you consider how to make use of the full range of the P.I.E.S.S. in your care recipient's leisure time and for your own life balance too.

Some leisure activities fit neatly into one or another category of the P.I.E.S.S., while many others overlap several areas. Dancing, for example, has both physical and self-expressive dimensions and might also produce spiritual or social outcomes for participants. The chapters of this book are organized according to the P.I.E.S.S. of Activities. Although there is some overlap among the P.I.E.S.S., and the activities discussed in each chapter may have a variety of outcomes, the activities are placed in the chapter that is most closely related to the primary outcome of that activity.

The "expected outcomes" of activities is a term that refers to what benefit we can hope to derive from participating in activities. Perhaps you never thought about why you do certain activities, but it is useful for all of us to analyze our leisure activities in relation to their expected outcomes. We may not even realize that activities have structures, rules, and required actions that affect us in many ways. These elements often explain why we enjoy certain activities and don't care for others. Some activities meet our needs. Others do not. Think about your usual leisure activities and what you have to gain by participating in them.

Consider, too, how specific activities might benefit the person you are caring for, by thinking through their expected outcomes.

When we understand the expected outcomes of leisure activities, we can do them for all the right reasons. For example, if I am feeling lonely and want to talk to someone, I need to choose an activity that has interaction built into it rather than going to a movie with someone and sitting side by side never saying a word. (Having coffee after the movie and talking about the movie would give me opportunity for the interaction I needed.) If I have been sitting most of the day, physical activity such as a brisk walk will provide the needed counterbalance, but watching TV all evening would not. We can make useful choices when we know the expected outcomes of activities.

In the P.I.E.S.S. chart below, you will find a list of some of the expected outcomes in each area. (Portions of this chart are used throughout the book to help you keep in mind the potential outcomes leisure activities offer.) As you plan leisure activities, consider how you can help the person in your care, as well as yourself, develop useful expected outcomes related to the P.I.E.S.S.

P.I.E.S.S.: *The Benefits of Leisure Activities*

Here are some of the benefits of

☆ *Physical* activities: balance, coordination, endurance, flexibility, strength, circulation enhancement, increased oxygen intake, decreased fatigue, weight control.

☆ *Intellectual* activities enable one to maintain listening and speaking skills, pay attention, learn, make decisions, recognize, recall, reminisce, follow directions, judge, match, strategize; they also help with reality orientation and stimulation of the senses.

☆ *Emotional/Expressive* activities offer the opportunity for variety of expressions and moods and allow one to feel and express feelings and individuality, increase self-esteem, take risks, feel consequences, and have fun!

☆ *Social* activities can put one in contact with people, plants, pets, the community, and provide occasions to meet people, talk, share interests, make and nurture relationships, join in activities, and build group cohesiveness.

☆ *Spiritual* activities make it possible to be in touch with one's Higher Power, express personal beliefs and values, collect thoughts, meditate, contemplate life and death, manage stress, appreciate beauty and life, and feel uplifted, motivated, inspired.

Finding Leisure Patterns

We know we like certain leisure activities and don't like others. We generally make time to do our favorite things and are too busy for those we dislike. Our favorite sports, games, places, music, books, movies, and snacks give us the starting point for a good time. I call "favorites" the "hot buttons" because they put "get up and go" into us even when we're tired, grumpy, or overworked. A person who is refusing to play cards may get up and go if you mention cribbage. Someone else may doze while classical music plays, but when it's their favorite Big Band tape, they get up and dance. When the topic turns to hunting, it may be difficult to get a word in with a formerly silent dinner partner. The "hot buttons" are favorites that *naturally* motivate us to participate.

Another way to think about the hot buttons might be to consider what makes a person happy. In her book called *14,000 Things to Be Happy About*, Barbara Ann Kipfer lists the things that made her happy over a period of twenty years. In her view, happiness comes from noticing and enjoying the little things in life. Her list is a reminder of just how many things can—and do—make us happy. She says, "Sometimes, on a gray day, I flip through this collection to cheer myself up; often I use it to get ideas about what to cook for dinner or something fun to do with my son on the weekend." You may find her system useful for both you and the person in your care. Keeping track of what makes your care receiver happy may be another good way to identify the favorites that you can use to brighten the days and plan meaningful activities.

What is enjoyable to one person, however, may be frustrating to another. It's important to know the person in order to understand what will motivate him or her to get involved in activities you plan. And, if you know past leisure patterns, you'll find it easier to know what to do for meaningful moments. It is important to avoid going by stereotypes or by what others think. Not all men enjoy sports; not all women want to sew. We cannot assume to know what someone else likes or dislikes, even when we've known that person for a long time, so we may as well have some fun finding those "hot buttons."

Gathering Information

You can consider yourself an "investigator of fun" in the other person's life. Find out what she or he liked (and still likes) to do, when, where, how often, with whom. Here are some strategies to use to help you obtain such information.

Visit with the person. Make it a real two-way exchange. Don't just pump someone with questions. Instead, have some fun talking about activities you enjoy, and see if you strike common ground. If I tell you that I grew up on a farm, gardened with my mother, and now enjoy my own garden vegetables and flowers, we already have something to talk about. You can tell me where you grew up, whether or not you know anything about gardening, and whether you like vegetables, flowers, or both. Visiting is a two-way street that is enjoyable in itself and can reveal information about the other person's leisure patterns. It may also help you understand your own leisure habits better, and it will definitely help you develop social skills throughout your life, not just in your caregiving situation.

Ask questions and move conversations toward memories of fun times. When you ask questions about leisure pursuits, you are showing interest in the person. Listen for clues about what the person enjoyed in the past. Through your questions, move the conversation toward good memories. Reminiscing, discussed in detail in Chapter 4, is an enjoyable activity in itself. It is also a way to gather information about leisure interests. Encourage the person to tell you stories about leisure pursuits and special events in the "old days," whether they were last week or several years ago. Get into the stories. Find out exactly what went on during the good times, and note how you might bring some of those positive feelings into current activities.

Observe what the person was doing in photos that may be in albums or around the house. You may find photos of the person on fishing trips, posing with baked goods or craft items, singing, or dancing. These are important guides to use in planning leisure possibilities now.

Get clues from the items in the home, if possible. Such things as handmade pillow tops, a collection of favorite music, woodworking tools, special-interest magazines, fishing gear, table games, puzzles, maps, and wall hangings can really help you get to know the person and his or her interests.

Conversations with family members, friends, neighbors, or health-care workers may also provide clues about past leisure habits. You may uncover details and insights to round out the other information you have. In situations where the person receiving your care is not able to communicate, the family may be your only source of information. If family members are not available to give such information, you may need to use a "trial and error" method of engaging the person in an activity and closely observing his or her responses. Observe what brings a smile and participation and what leads to a frown or the end of action. Overall, leisure patterns continue over a lifetime. People who love to socialize generally continue to enjoy being with other people, while "loners" do not suddenly become socialites. Those who were physically active in their youth tend to maintain interest in physical activity as long as health allows, while those who preferred passive activities are inclined to remain more passive as they age. This doesn't mean that a person cannot change; but, overall, daily joys are more likely to come from the activities a person always knew and enjoyed.

The Checklist of Leisure Favorites

The Checklist of Leisure Favorites presented on the following pages will help you get an overview of a person's leisure needs and interests. (Use it to check on your own interests and patterns, too.) My suggestion is for you to go over the Checklist, a little at a time, with the person in your care. If you do this gently and leisurely, you can turn the process itself into a leisure activity. Have some fun with it! For instance, you might use the first section, on general favorites, as a conversation starter or as the basis for reminiscing and telling stories. In fact, just asking someone what he prefers to be called may lead to an hour's worth of stories about nicknames! Remember, the whole process should be enjoyable for both of you. There's no point in adding to your burden.

There is no time limit on gathering this information. It might take several conversations or even a few weeks. As with anything in life, attitude matters. If you approach the Checklist with a negative attitude, it's not as likely to be enjoyable for you or the other person. On the other hand, if you take your time and go through a piece of the Checklist one day and talk about a different section another day, you will have a chance to discuss leisure activities in many ways and on different occasions. It doesn't matter how many conversations it takes, you can enjoy the process all along the way and begin to apply information as you get it.

Let the Checklist be a starting point for finding those "hot buttons" and planning ahead for fun activities. If you are a volunteer or a part-time caregiver, you can use the Checklist as a source of conversation topics to get to know the person. If you are one of several caregivers serving as a team, each of you might add to the Checklist as you gather information, using the tool as a central place to record information so you can all refer to it for ideas.

Don't "bug" the person about answering the Checklist of Leisure Favorites just to fill in the blanks. And don't feel as if you have to fill in the form in the order it appears here. It's better if you gather information in a way that is natural to your relationship. This is a case where you will want to fill in what you can and otherwise leave blank spaces. Just because you leave some blank spaces doesn't mean you haven't gathered information. Focus on what you do learn about the person's leisure and go from there.

The Checklist of Leisure Favorites

Name _____   Date begun _____

GENERAL FAVORITES (fill in the blanks):

Name (prefers to be called): _____

Family Members: _____
_____

Friends: _____
_____

Foods: _____
_____

Recipes: _____
_____

Beverages: _____
_____

Music: _____
_____

Songs: _____
_____

Books: _____
_____

Stories: _____
_____

Poems: _____
_____

Ethnic Traditions: _____
_____

TV Programs: _____

_____

Radio Programs: _____

_____

Movies: _____

_____

Videos: _____

_____

Actors: _____

_____

Actresses: _____

_____

Colors: _____

Seasons: _____

Hobbies: _____

_____

Games: _____

_____

Table Games: _____

Sports: _____

_____

Places: _____

_____

Parks or Campgrounds: _____

_____

Computer Activities: _____

_____

Electronic Equipment: _____

_____

Other: _____

_____

SCHEDULE PREFERENCES (check all of the following that apply):

_____ Early riser

_____ Late riser

_____ Likes to go to bed early

_____ Likes to stay up late

_____ No regular pattern of rising and retiring

PHYSICAL ACTIVITY FAVORITES (check those done in the past *and* those still possible; use the lines to record details about specific activities):

Past   Still Possible

_____ exercise routine   _____

                            _____

_____ walking   _____

                            _____

_____ running   _____

                            _____

_____ biking   _____

                            _____

_____ hiking   _____

                            _____

_____ dancing   _____

                            _____

_____ camping   _____

_____

_____ playing sports   _____

_____

_____ making love   _____

_____

REGARDING GENERAL BODY MOVEMENT (circle all that are still possible):

Related to Self-care

comb hair, put on shoes, reach for clothing, dress self, take shower,

take bath, other: _____

_____

Related to Household Chores

take out garbage, dust furniture, sweep floor, vacuum, care for plants,

do laundry, fold laundry, put away clean laundry, wash windows,

other: _____

Related to Meal Preparation

set the table, pour beverages, peel potatoes, peel other vegetables or

fruits, reach for items in cupboards, put away items in cupboards,

wipe table and/or cupboard tops, other: _____

_____

Related to Outdoors

mow grass, shovel or sweep sidewalk, rake, work in garden, care for

pets, take a walk on deck, take a walk on patio, take a walk in yard,

other: _____

_____

INTELLECTUAL ACTIVITY FAVORITES (check those done in the past *and* those still possible; use the lines to record details about specific activities):

Past   Still Possible

____ puzzles   _____

                                  _____

____ crossword puzzles   _____

                                  _____

____ mind-teasers   _____

                                  _____

____ table games   _____

                                  _____

____ reading   _____
      newspapers
                                  _____

____ reading   _____
      magazines
                                  _____

____ reading books   _____

                                  _____

____ reading poetry   _____

                                  _____

____ other reading   _____

                                  _____

____ listening to/   _____
      watching news
      programs   _____

                                  _____

____ listening to/   _____
      watching inform-
      ative programs   _____

                                  _____

_____ taking classes/
learning things

_____ working on
the computer

_____ communicating
electronically
(e-mail; Internet)

_____ writing letters

_____ writing a
personal
journal

_____ writing diary

_____ writing poetry

_____ other writing

_____ teaching

_____ telling stories
or jokes

_____ reminiscing

_____ other

FAVORITE EMOTIONAL/EXPRESSIVE ACTIVITIES AND HOBBIES (check those done in the past *and* those still possible; use the lines to record details about specific activities):

Past   Still Possible

____ jokes, humor   _____

                             _____

____ singing   _____

                             _____

____ dancing   _____

                             _____

____ playing   _____
     musical
     instrument   _____

                             _____

____ making love   _____

                             _____

____ acting   _____

                             _____

____ painting   _____

                             _____

____ drawing   _____

                             _____

____ arts and crafts   _____

                             _____

____ sewing   _____

                             _____

____ cooking   _____

                             _____

                             _____

_____ growing
vegetables

_____

_____

_____ growing flowers

_____

_____

_____ raising
house plants

_____

_____

_____ photography

_____

_____

_____ collecting things

_____

_____

_____ building things

_____

_____

_____ making things

_____

_____

_____ community
service

_____

_____

_____ other hobbies

_____

_____

FAVORITE SOCIAL ACTIVITIES WITH FAMILY, FRIENDS, AND OTHER
LIVING THINGS (check those that apply and use the lines to record details about specific activities):

Living family members: _____

_____

Nearby family members: _____

_____

Family members still able and willing to visit: _____

_____

"Best" friends: _____

_____

Friends still able and willing to visit: _____

_____

Entertained friends in the home: Often ____ Seldom ____ Never ____

Visited friends' homes: Often ____ Seldom ____ Never ____

Could still visit these friends' homes: _____

_____

Used to go out with friends: Often ____ Seldom ____ Never ____

Could still go out with friends to do: _____

_____

Likes to reminisce and tell stories: Often ____ Seldom ____ Never ____

Likes to play cards/table games with others:

Often ____ Seldom ____ Never ____

Other activities possible with family and friends now: _____

_____

_____

Regarding contact with living things and the wider community:

Enjoys pets: No ____ Yes ____

Which ones? _____

_____

Enjoys plants: No ____ Yes ____

Which ones? _____

_____

Enjoys watching people: No ____ Yes ____

Enjoys being with children: No ____ Yes ____

Enjoys talking on the phone: No _____ Yes _____

Enjoys talking on e-mail or the Internet: No _____ Yes _____

Enjoys membership in clubs and organizations: No _____ Yes _____

Which? _____

Enjoys leadership roles in the community: No _____ Yes _____

Which? _____

Enjoys being alone: No _____ Yes _____

Other favorite social experiences: _____

_____

_____

HOLIDAY FAVORITES (fill in the blanks):

Favorite Holidays: _____

How celebrated: _____

_____

_____

Special traditions: _____

_____

_____

Traditions to keep or add now: _____

_____

_____

Special people usually present: _____

_____

_____

Who to celebrate with now? _____

_____

REGARDING OUTINGS (check those done in the past *and* those still possible; use the lines to record details about specific activities):

Past   Still Possible

____ go for a walk
in the yard

____ go for a walk
in the
neighborhood

____ go for a car ride

____ go for a bus ride

____ visit home of
family member

____ visit home of
friend or
neighbor

____ go out for a meal

____ go out for a
snack

____ go to church,
temple, or
synagogue

____ go to sporting
events

_____ go to movies

_____

_____

_____ go to concerts

_____

_____

_____ go to plays

_____

_____

_____ go shopping

_____

_____

_____ go to the park

_____

_____

_____ go camping

_____

_____

_____ day trip

_____

_____

_____ weekend trip

_____

_____

_____ "armchair travel"
(watching video-
tapes of places of

_____

interest, such as:)

_____

_____ other

_____

FAVORITE SPIRITUAL ACTIVITIES (check all desired):

Enjoys spiritual reading materials: Often _____ Seldom _____ Never _____
(Examples: scripture, Great Books, poetry, inspirational stories, motivational materials, photography books, art books, music books)

Favorites: _____

_____

Engage in prayer: Often _____ Seldom _____ Never _____

Favorites: _____

_____

Attend religious services: Often _____ Seldom _____ Never _____

Visit with minister or rabbi: Often _____ Seldom _____ Never _____

Participate in socials at church, temple, or synagogue:

Often _____ Seldom _____ Never _____

Visits from people of church, temple, synagogue:

Often _____ Seldom _____ Never _____

Listen to or watch religious services on radio, TV:

Often _____ Seldom _____ Never _____

Favorites: _____

_____

Listen to tapes of religious services:

Often _____ Seldom _____ Never _____

Enjoy nature walks, gardens, woods:

Often _____ Seldom _____ Never _____

Enjoy camping, the wilderness: Often _____ Seldom _____ Never _____

Visit inspirational places: Often _____ Seldom _____ Never _____

Favorites: _____

_____

Enjoy comforting, inspirational music:

Often _____ Seldom _____ Never _____

Favorites: _____

_____

Listen to/watch inspirational radio, TV programs:

Often _____ Seldom _____ Never _____

Favorites: _____

_____

Listen to inspirational audiotapes:

Often ____ Seldom ____ Never ____

Favorites: _____

_____

Watch inspirational videotapes: Often ____ Seldom ____ Never ____

Favorites: _____

_____

Contemplate/Meditate: Often ____ Seldom ____ Never ____

Do Yoga: Often ____ Seldom ____ Never ____

Keep a personal journal: No ____ Yes ____

Just be quiet: Often ____ Seldom ____ Never ____

Other: _____

_____

_____

Summary of Leisure Favorites

General favorites: _____

_____

_____

_____

Favorite physical activities: _____

_____

_____

Favorite intellectual activities: _____

_____

_____

Favorite expressive activities and hobbies: _____

_____

_____

Favorite social activities: _____

_____

_____

Favorite spiritual activities: _____

_____

_____

After gathering this information regarding leisure patterns in the person's life, make realistic, simplified plans for ongoing, meaningful activity. The next five chapters will give you many activity ideas, and Chapter 8 offers planning strategies that will help you plan specific activities.

Summary

The P.I.E.S.S. System of behavioral domains refers to the physical, intellectual, emotional/expressive, social, and spiritual behaviors involved in leisure activities. This system offers a useful way to think about the benefits we can hope to derive from participating in activities. Everyone has leisure favorites, and when we know what someone likes to do, it is easier to plan activities that are naturally motivating to that person. Use the Checklist of Leisure Favorites as a starting point to get to know a person's leisure patterns. Take your time; gather information gradually. It is likely a person receiving care will not be able to give you all the information asked on the Checklist—*especially* at one time. Just gather what you can and begin to use it. Collect additional information through observation, visiting, and reminiscence. Make the information-gathering process enjoyable for both of you!

CHAPTER THREE

Physical Activity

BENEFITS
Physical activities can give one balance, coordination, endurance, flexibility, strength, circulation enhancement, increased oxygen intake, decreased fatigue, weight control.

In Chapters 1 and 2 we laid the foundation for understanding leisure, its importance in caregiving, and for the physical, intellectual, emotional, social, and spiritual benefits we can expect from participating in leisure activities. Now, we will begin to look at specific types of activities and how to use them. In this chapter you will find a discussion of the following:

☆ The importance of physical activity
☆ Stories describing how to blend general body movement into leisure and daily living
☆ Guidelines for age-appropriate activity
☆ Ideas for making useful modifications so the activities will suit the person

A friend of mine is very good at reminding himself to stay active in his later years just as he did throughout his life. He begins his day with stretches before leaving his bed and he walks for twenty to thirty minutes before breakfast. He takes his wife and friends with him and enjoys this social start to his day while reaping the benefits in good health. After short, rapid walks, many people feel more optimistic, and personal problems appear less serious. There are so many positive outcomes from simple walking that it is a wonder we aren't *all* doing more of it. It may be because we dislike the idea of exercise and associate it with pain and discomfort. However, exercise and movement can be a natural part of leisure activities and therefore can be done in a context of enjoyment rather than pain. The key is to find physical activity we *enjoy* and do it regularly. If we don't enjoy it, we likely will not do it. Only an exercise program that is enjoyable will last—and *work*. Walking the dog, gardening, shooting baskets, bowling, walking in the woods, chopping wood, mowing the lawn, biking, hiking, swimming— do whatever you *enjoy*, and it will not seem like exercise, yet you will gain the benefits.

Even small amounts of physical activity can benefit both body and mind. Physical recreation activities are generally more motivating than routine calisthenics, and they also contribute to muscular strength, cardiovascular fitness, vital capacity, flexibility, and balance. It is beneficial for everyone, caregivers and care receivers alike, to remain active and engage in physical activity to whatever extent is possible.

In this chapter I am not recommending high-level physical exercise or a regimen of heavy workouts. Instead, the idea here is that simple, natural body movement can be pleasurable and, at the same time, contribute to health and peace of mind. Most of the activities suggested here promote simple body movement blended with enjoyment. These activities should not bring pain or distress to the person in your care. Rather, they should be naturally enjoyable. To assure that the physical activities you do with your care receiver are suited to his or her needs, you may want to consult with a health professional. Your care receiver's doctor is likely to know what the person can or can't do, and will be able to advise you about movements that are useful. A physical therapist or a professional who specializes in exercise also could be of help. Together, you can look for ways to blend easy, natural movement into the daily activities of the person in your care, and focus on "feeling good" and maintaining good health. The following stories will give you ideas for blending movement into daily living.

General Body Movement

William

William showed signs of confusion. Family members tried to spend late afternoon and evening hours with him. Diane, his granddaughter, volunteered to spend one evening a week with William. Because the doctor had encouraged family members to keep William as active as possible, in little ways, since he had a tendency to just sit, Diane decided she would try to make the time useful to William's physical well-being, and try to have a little fun, too. It wasn't calisthenics or physical therapy she had in mind. Just a little wiggle now and then.

Diane did some creative thinking about how she could include simple physical activity into William's evening. At supper time, she made the meal preparation into a team effort. When she asked for his help and worked *with* him, she found that he would help to set the table, reach into cupboards for plates, cups, glasses, and walk to the drawer for silverware and back to the table to complete the place settings. They talked while they worked, and she gave William verbal praise for his help, saying things like, "I appreciate your help." "This goes better when we work together." The attention she gave him during their work seemed to be the encouragement he needed to participate. The stretching, carrying, and walking, though minimal, were at least *some* movement in his day.

Diane knew that her grandfather often had played catch after supper with his own children when they were growing up. Now, it seemed natural when Diane wanted to play catch with him. She used a beach ball, though, and they threw it back and forth in the living room where William sat in his lounge chair. This activity involved bending, throwing, grasping, and reaching. When weather permitted, they sat on the porch for the ball games. Diane noticed they both laughed and teased while they played catch. William seemed less confused when they laughed. Diane also found the physical activity section of the Checklist of Leisure Favorites helpful in assessing William's physical activity. She made it a point to tell other family members about the success she had in helping him to be a little more active, and she explained her strategies so they could do some physical activities with him when they were "on duty."

Just by helping to get things ready for supper, William had a chance to move and get some exercise without even knowing it. Diane used natural movements as exercise for him. Walking across the room, across the porch, or across the backyard is considered natural movement for someone able to walk. What feels like natural lifting, stretching, bending, pushing, and pulling will vary according to the person's health and level of fitness. As health changes, you can make adjustments in the activities you use. Movement must fit the person's abilities or disabilities.

General body movement is the kind of movement we do in the course of our daily living. It is an important form of physical exercise even though it is not done solely for the sake of physical benefit, but rather because we move to complete some task. It is what we do when we garden, climb the stairs, dress ourselves, sweep the floor, wash dishes. Allowing your care receiver to do whatever is still possible such as lifting items into cupboards, stretching to open a window, or bending to tie shoes will give him or her a good opportunity for general body movement.

If someone is confined to bed, in a weak or deteriorating condition due to cancer or other progressive disease, there still are ways to encourage general body movement. When you pull the drapes to allow in sunshine, help the person roll over to see out the window or to feel the warmth of the sun. Squeezing a plush animal, a soft rubber ball, or a piece of foam rubber is comforting to some people and also provides a small amount of general body movement when physical abilities are severely limited.

To promote stretching, find a length of elastic (one-quarter to one-half inch wide) in your sewing box, or buy one at the notions counter of a store. Tie together the two ends of a comfortable length (two or three feet) to form an expandable loop that your care receiver can hold to stretch arms and hands. Or, hold on to the loop with the other person and together enjoy the push and pull of the elastic in various directions, high and low. You will both get some exercise, and you will feel each other's movements in a nonverbal communication that feels good and often brings a smile. If elastic is not available, nylon stockings have similar elastic qualities and can serve well for stretching purposes.

It is important never to force movement or allow strain. Let the person take the lead in determining what movement feels comfortable or how much is enough. Be observant and be sure movement is not causing strain and discomfort. Because we are talking about general body movement here, "gentle" and "comfortable" are the key words to keep in mind for healthful movement.

You can have some fun building physical movement into daily routines. Be creative and plan ahead for blending physical movement into ordinary activities. This is a good idea for yourself as well as for your care receiver. For instance, when you are out parking your car, don't look for the closest parking space. Rather, find a space that gives you more distance to walk; enjoy the fresh air while getting the exercise you designed for yourself on the way to your destination. When you watch TV, put away the remote control and get up to change the channels or volume. Does this sound like an old-fashioned idea? It may be, but it will get you moving.

So, too, you can find ways to involve the person receiving care in daily activities such as food preparation and moving around a room, the house, or yard. If you have a habit of doing everything for your care receiver, think about how you can encourage more independence and more physical movement. If he or she is able to bend, stop yourself from picking up everything that falls; allow time for him or her to reach for bowls of food on the table rather than doing it first, even if it takes a little longer. Even those small movements are important. Every little bit counts and helps to maintain abilities and strength.

If you are a friendly visitor, whether a friend or a volunteer, find ways to bring movement into the visit. If the person you are visiting walks or uses a wheelchair to meet you at the door, you might prolong that movement before sitting down by suggesting a look out the window to see the rain or snow, the birds, or new leaves on the trees. Even a walk across the room like that will be additional general body movement in the person's day.

Movement to Music

Arlene

Arlene, diagnosed with dementia, was being cared for by her daughter Dell and her family. Dell realized her mother was becoming more and more lethargic, sitting long hours in an easy chair or lying in bed for long periods of the day. Dell did what she could, though, to help her mother stay alert and get a little movement into her routine.

Arlene had always enjoyed music from the "big band" era, and Dell played those records and tapes for her mother from time to time. Arlene's dementia didn't keep her from humming the tunes and even chiming in some words here and there. One day Dell put on a Glenn

Miller tape and sat in front of her mother. She pretended to be directing the band while she sang along, and soon Arlene started "directing"
too. Dell used the opportunity to have Arlene follow her movements,
which she exaggerated into high, low, and wide beats to the music. Arlene mirrored her daughter's movements while she enjoyed the familiar music.

Many afternoons after school, Dell's eight-year-old daughter,
Heather, spent time with Grandma and discovered that Arlene enjoyed
hitting a balloon back and forth. She would reach and stretch to return
the balloon to Heather. Dell's daughter also enjoyed blowing bubbles
with her grandmother. Arlene naturally hit the bubbles, had a few
laughs with Heather, and got a little exercise in the process.

Arlene seemed to automatically move when the music played. Both
she and her daughter had fun while getting a little exercise. Movement
to music is natural and easy. When we like the music, it seems like the
thing to do—tap our feet, move our arms, and keep the beat. It is best
to use the care receiver's favorite music if possible. (The Checklist of
Leisure Favorites will help you find the favorites.) Of course, any music may do, but a person is more apt to move to his or her *favorite* music. The person is likely to respond best if you do the movements and
have him or her follow you. Better yet, get up and dance if possible. If
you feel uncomfortable with this at first, try to keep a light, humorous
attitude and be willing to laugh at yourself; you can giggle while you
move. That will serve as additional exercise for both of you. (I've heard
laughter described as "inner jogging.")

Keeping time to music is an activity well suited to a person who has
dementia, since the person's sense of rhythm and movement usually
remains intact. If the person in your care has cognitive impairment,
think of ways to blend rhythmic activities into daily living. Dancing,
rocking, folding, sawing, and sanding will feel natural to the person
and also provide for healthy movement. Arlene's granddaughter added
the child's touch of fun to her movement, but we don't have to have
children around to encourage exercise through playful activity. Batting
a beach ball, hitting bubbles in the air, tossing a nerf ball, playing catch
with a rolled-up sock are easy-to-do activities that can provide general
body movement and help keep a person more alert. A word of caution
about balloons: be sure to pick up and discard all pieces of broken bal-

loons to prevent people or pets in the household from swallowing them and choking.

Guidelines for Age-Appropriate Activity

Balloons, bubbles, nerf balls, and other toys and certain games bring up the issue of the age appropriateness of items and activities we use with those in our care. I believe some items are "ageless" in their potential for usefulness and fun. I think that balloons are "ageless," and that the person who invented them should have received a Nobel Peace Prize, because people of all ages smile and laugh over balloons. Not everyone agrees with me, though, and some adults are offended when asked to play with balloons, thinking of them as being for children only. It is important, for this issue as for others, to know your care receiver and be alert to his or her responses in order to prevent giving offense of any kind.

It is also important to prevent situations where outsiders might ridicule or give negative attention to a person because they consider an activity to be childish. Some people take offense when they see adults playing with items they consider to be children's toys or see them engaged in activities generally considered to be for children. The following guidelines for age appropriateness will be helpful in deciding what does or does not suit the situation.

To help determine whether or not an item or an activity is age appropriate, use these two guidelines: (1) If other people you know of the same age generally use the item or do the activity, it is age appropriate. If, on the other hand, people you know of the same age would receive negative attention or be ridiculed for using the item or doing the activity, it may not be appropriate for that person in a public situation. (2) The second guideline regarding age appropriateness, then, relates to where the activity takes place. In private, whatever is comfortable and comforting is age appropriate. In public you need to take other people's potential reactions into account. For example, in my own home no one knows or cares if I play with a baby's rattle or hold and talk to a teddy bear while I watch TV. I may find those activities comforting. In my home, what I do is my business. However, if I play with a baby's rattle while I teach a class or talk to a teddy bear when I shop for groceries, I am subjecting myself to the negative attention of others. I would hope someone who cares for me would stop me from being in that situation. Negative attention can be damaging to a person's emotional well-being. As the provider of care, you can protect the other person from such uncomfortable situations by applying the guidelines for age appropriateness stated above.

Modifying Activities

Josh

Following diagnosis of progressive cancer, Josh, twenty-three, lived at home with his parents, who shared caregiving responsibilities along with home-health aides. He was able to be up in a lounge chair on some days but remained in bed to rest other days. He was easily bored with TV and missed his previous active lifestyle which included a variety of sports. He enjoyed the company of friends who visited, especially Marco. When Marco came, they reminisced about ball games and dart games and shooting baskets in the backyard.

One afternoon when Josh bragged about his great hook shot, he squashed a piece of paper and tossed it at the wastebasket to emphasize his story, and that gave Marco an idea. He brought the wastebasket into a convenient place for both of them to play "wastebasket ball" and rolled several of Josh's socks to use as the "balls." They made up their own rules, kept score, and carried on the game as though it were for a championship. All their laughter brought Josh's dad to the room, and of course he had to play, too. From then on, when Marco visited, they played their indoor "sports." He brought a set of chips usually used for card games and they shot them one by one into different sized plastic bowls, and he found a small dart board with velcro-tipped darts so they could shoot darts in Josh's room. Their games simulated the sports they had enjoyed together for years, and provided some physical movement which Josh needed. Even when he was having a bad day, he perked up when Marco arrived for a game or two. It gave them both something to look forward to and something to do during visits. The scores posted on Josh's wall kept their competitive spirits ready for the next game.

It is possible to modify activities to include familiar movements. The modified indoor "sports" Josh and Marco shared were far less sophisticated than their earlier "real" sports experiences, but the indoor games they created had familiar movements, rules, and competition. If your care receiver likes sports and games, see how you can make up related activities to promote physical activity.

On the other hand, be aware that sometimes people want to do the "real thing" or nothing at all. Josh and Marco seemed to find enjoyment in the competitive pastime they dreamed up, but other people may think such games are fake, or childish. Competition, too, may be motivating to some but not to others. It may take a trial and error approach to discover someone's opinions on such matters. If one thing doesn't work, try another. Don't be discouraged by refusal. Keep trying to find the "hot buttons" (discussed in Chapter 1).

Modifying games and activities can be fun in itself. You will have the best results if you involve the other person as much as possible in trying to figure out exactly how to modify an activity so it is fun and interesting. Have some fun making possible changes that work. Children are very good at doing this. If you listen to them on the playground, you will hear them suggesting one change after another. "Let's do it this way, then I'll do this and you do that. Okay?" Sometimes playmates go along with suggestions, sometimes not. It is common, though, for adults to lose that kind of flexibility in their "play." Sports and recreational pursuits often have rules and specified tasks leaving little room to make things up along the way. When illness and disability come into the picture, however, modifications and adaptations may be necessary if there is to be any participation at all. You can have a good time rediscovering the natural talent you had as a child, to make things up as you go. In leisure, it's not only acceptable but *the thing to do*.

Perhaps the person in your care needs special equipment to participate in certain sports or games. Adapted devices such as battery-operated fishing reels with automatic cast and reel-in options and bowling balls with retractable handles for whole-hand grip of the ball allow many people to enjoy leisure activities they would otherwise have to discontinue. For information about adapted devices, you might contact companies that specialize in adapted recreation equipment (some are listed in the Related Resources section of this book), or a sporting goods store may refer you to a supplier. Or, contact a therapeutic recreation specialist at a health-care agency in your area. He or she can provide information on where to obtain adapted devices or can help you modify existing equipment for successful participation.

Adding Interest to Physical Movement
Gerard

After his stroke and ensuing rehabilitation, Gerard lived in an assisted living arrangement and had volunteer visitors three afternoons each week. Using a cane, Gerard was able to walk slowly, though with a shuffle. Keiko volunteered to take Gerard for afternoon walks and tried to make them interesting besides useful as exercise. To motivate Gerard to get out of his room and into the fresh air, she invited him to go with her on a "snoop walk." They looked for specific things along their route. They snooped into the janitor's workshop down the hall from Gerard's room and looked at brooms and buckets there, they snooped outside for dandelions, checked behind the building and into an empty barrel, looked through a garage window to see what they could see, crossed the street to the park to snoop into the flower gardens, and tried to find large black stones. Keiko managed to occupy Gerard's mind while he walked for physical exercise; she kept him curious about what might come next. They did a lot of reminiscing on their walks, too. So many things they found led to stories and good talks. They both enjoyed their walks. Not only did Gerard get involved in "snooping," but he always reached for his cane as soon as he saw Keiko come to his door.

Keiko seemed to know how to blend variety into activities to get Gerard out of his room to walk. You, too, can find ways to combine other ideas with physical movement for motivation and added interest. In this case, Keiko created a mental game, "snooping," that promoted Gerard's physical movement. A "snoop walk" is especially suitable for persons who are curious and who can understand and make appropriate responses. If the person in your care might improperly carry the idea of snooping into other daily living, then give your walking time a different title, such as "walk about and talk about" (while you walk, talk about things you see) or "walk around and look around" (look at things along the walking trail). These titles carry the same idea—doing something *along with* walking. Walks like these can take place anytime and almost anywhere: indoors, in a house, in just one room, in a mall, a store, a park, a neighborhood, or backyard. Be creative and see how much bending, reaching, stretching, and walking you can build into a "snoop walk" that suits you and the other person. If using a wheelchair, snoop for things that require bending and reaching from the chair; have the other person give directions about where to go and what to look for. Take enough time to enjoy things along the way that will add interest and overall refreshment. Use opportunities to *truly* smell the flowers you find, delight in the play of children, and enjoy fragrances, colors, sounds, and conversations as opportunities arise. The idea is not only to build movement into the day to get some exercise, but to make the moments count.

Summary

As leisure experience, physical movement can be both enjoyable and beneficial for physical, mental, and emotional health. When we exercise through enjoyable activities we are likely to continue the activities and thereby gain ongoing benefits. General body movement is a basic form of exercise which can be blended into activities of daily living and a variety of nontraditional leisure activities. For optimal health and stress management, both caregivers and care receivers need to remain as physically active as conditions allow, even in the midst of the caregiving process.

Physical Activity Ideas Related to General Body Movement

care for plants or pets	clean cupboards
comb hair	do laundry
dress self	dust furniture
fold laundry	hang decorations
make love	mow grass
peel vegetables	pour beverages
pull taffy	put away clean laundry
put on shoes	rake
reach for clothing	reach items in cupboard
rearrange furniture	set the table

string beads or buttons
stretch a nylon stocking
squeeze a plush animal
sweep the sidewalk
take out the garbage
unpack groceries
wind yarn into a ball

stretch elastic
squeeze a foam ball
sweep the floor
take a bath
wash the windows
vacuum the carpet
take a walk—to the next room, to the
    porch, around the block, or in the yard

other _____   _____

Ideas Related to Sports, Games, and Exercise

bike
breathe deeply
dance
fly paper airplanes
hit a balloon in the air
move to music
pitch pennies
play catch
play frisbee
play indoor bowling
play "Twister"
shoot baskets
stack blocks
toss a beach ball
toss things into a basket

bounce a ball
chase butterflies
do chair exercises
hike
kick a can
lift arms and legs
play badminton
play darts
play golf
play pool
shake dice
skip stones
stretch
toss rings over bottles
walk

other _____   _____

CHAPTER FOUR

Intellectual Activity

BENEFITS

Intellectual activities help one to maintain listening and speaking skills, pay attention, learn, make decisions, recognize, recall, reminisce, follow directions, judge, match, strategize; also help with reality orientation and stimulation of the senses.

Moving along through the P.I.E.S.S.—from physical to intellectual activities—we will see in this chapter that there are many interesting yet simple ways to combine leisure and mental stimulation. Your care recipient's mental abilities may not allow participation in difficult activities but instead require simplification. This chapter offers ideas to help you modify and adapt activities to keep the mind active and have some fun, too. The chapter covers the following topics:

☆ How to keep the mind active
☆ Reality orientation
☆ Learning opportunities, television, and entertainment
☆ How to modify intellectual activities
☆ Recreational reminiscence
☆ Blending sensory stimulation into leisure activities and daily living

Keeping the Mind Active

Intellectual activities include paying attention, listening, speaking, using the memory, matching things, solving problems, following directions, strategizing, recalling, and making choices. All these mental actions are common to daily living and are built into leisure activities such as puzzles, table games, computer games, reminiscing, and reading the newspaper. Such leisure pursuits can be both enjoyable and useful in keeping the mind active. A 1991 study by leisure researchers Carol Riddick and M. Jean Keller showed that when participating in board games, video games, writing, reality orientation, and reminiscence, persons with dementia improved their intellectual functioning and memory. Those activities also showed a positive impact on life satisfaction, mood, and leisure experience among the participants. Such research shows that intellectual activities are powerful tools for both fun and mental development, and well worth some effort to make them available to a person receiving care.

Orienting for Reality

"Reality orientation" refers to a person's awareness of his or her environment and includes knowing such things as where one is; the time of day; week, month, and season of the year; weather conditions; upcoming holidays; and the names of people who are present. The reality orientation opportunities you provide for your care receiver will not require a structured program. Instead, through casual conversation and daily interactions you can keep the person informed about his or her environment. It can be as simple as including in conversation, clues about what is going on in household routines and in the day's schedule.

In the caregiving process, you are likely to find yourself following a schedule based on the needs of the person you care for. Night and day schedules get mixed up; eating, sleeping, getting up, engaging in conversation or activity may or may not follow the routines of the rest of the world. These daily activities take place when they best suit the needs at hand. You simply respond to needs as they arise and pay little or no attention to what is going on outside your enclosed world. In spite of the unique schedule you may follow, make it a point to give your care receiver clues about the reality of the immediate environment. You can do this in daily conversation, several times a day if that is suitable and useful. Here is a sample statement that shows how you might include reality orientation in general conversation: "Good morning, Jim. It's 8:00 in the morning. I'm your wife, Joanne, coming to wake you up so we can have breakfast together. It is Saturday, January twentieth, a cold winter day, and we have a little snow on the ground this morning. Tomorrow is your birthday, so let's make a cake later. I know how much you love chocolate cake." If possible, I would continue by opening the drape and looking at the weather conditions outdoors to allow Jim to make the connection between the information I gave him and the reality he can see through the window.

In this one bit of conversation, I gave Jim clues regarding (1) his name, (2) my name and relationship to him, (3) time of day, (4) month, (5) date, (6) day, (7) season of the year, (8) weather conditions outdoors, (9) a special event coming up tomorrow, (10) an activity to look forward to today, and (11) one of his favorite things. It is more important to give hints about the environment than to ask questions and put Jim on the spot as to what he knows or does not know, what he remembers or does not remember about his world. It may not matter to him whether it is Saturday or Thursday. He may or may not be able to participate in keeping track of the days of the week or a doctor's appointment scheduled for a specific time and day. Yet, I can give him information and try to keep him alert and in touch with his world. Depending on Jim's condition, I may continue to give reality clues in conversation throughout the day.

Remember, the goal here is to keep the mind active, not to test ability to remember information correctly. Perhaps a professional who would administer a test to your care receiver would ask reality orientation questions to seek information about his or her mental state. This is not your purpose. Rather, you can stimulate your care receiver's mind and provide a bridge to reality through hints and clues blended into conversation and daily experiences. Besides, it gives you something to talk about.

Learning New Things

Many people who need care and supervision can still enjoy learning new things. Educational opportunities are available even for people who are homebound, in that many community education and community service programs offer short courses on a variety of topics. We usually think that actually attending the course on location is required, but more and more programs are offering the option of having a caregiver or a volunteer attend the class for the person at home. In this "surrogate student" arrangement, the person attending class does so in the name of the other person who is homebound, and then teaches the content to the other at home. Some community education and community service programs offer educational materials and equipment on loan to those who are homebound. Art supplies, paintbrushes, adapted brushes, large-face playing cards, electric scissors, needlepoint hoops and grips, needle threaders, and videotapes often can be checked out for home use through some local community education or community services programs. If the person in your care has interest in educational activities and has special needs, call your local services and request the assistance you need.

Some care receivers have access to computers, e-mail, and the Internet, which provide new and interesting opportunities to keep the mind active. For some people the Internet provides a way of staying in touch with other people and the world. A friend of mine who is quadriplegic uses a mouth stick to operate his computer and spends hours each day on the Internet pursuing numerous areas of interest. He has even taken college courses by way of e-mail and Internet connections. Computer games also offer interesting intellectual activity for people of all ages. A 1991 study by therapeutic recreation specialist L. Peniston found that older people with mild and moderate memory loss who participated in a six-week computer game program demonstrated significant improvement in cognitive strategies, attention, memory, and impulse control when compared to a group without computer activity. If the person who is homebound has access to electronic equipment and computer activities and finds them interesting, do what you can to help him or her continue this important leisure pursuit.

Promoting Former Interests

How a person spends his or her leisure time says a lot about who that person is and what is most enjoyable in life. So that the person can continue to enjoy former interests that keep the mind active, you need to know how he or she spent leisure time in the past. The "intellectual activity" segment of the Checklist of Leisure Favorites will be helpful in finding those "hot buttons" related to a person's "old-favorite" intellectual leisure pursuits. The following sections describe some situations where people were able to accommodate activities so former interests could still be pursued.

Talking Books

Ginger

Since her stroke several months ago, Ginger has lost nearly all her vision, and now lives with her caregiving sister, Judith. Among other activities they enjoyed over the years, the sisters had been members of the same book club. They loved to read and discuss a variety of literature and poetry. By working through the Checklist of Leisure Favorites, Judith discovered Ginger missed reading more than anything else.

During her rehabilitation following the stroke, a vocational rehabilitation counselor told Ginger about a wide range of services for people who have visual and physical impairments. One of the things she learned was how she could continue to learn things by using a cassette player, ear phones, and Talking Books—cassette recordings of books and magazines. Judith helped Ginger to make the necessary contact with their state's regional library so they could obtain the required equipment and some cassettes to begin Ginger's new form of reading. Not only was Ginger able to enjoy listening to the same books Judith read, but they continued to discuss them as much as Ginger could these days. Judith also discovered, at a local book store, a few commercial tapes of old radio programs. Once in a while she and Ginger listened to old episodes of Jack Benny, Fibber McGee and Molly, and Baby Snooks. They enjoyed them, had some hearty laughs, and reminisced about growing up with the radio.

Because of her visual and physical limitations, Ginger qualified to receive many special services, which included Talking Books. Similarly, if your care receiver is having difficulty reading regular print, such as newspaper print, due to physical or visual impairment, he or she may qualify for adapted reading devices available through your state's services for people who are visually and physically impaired. Talking Books are complete audio renditions of bestsellers, classic books, poetry, scripture—almost anything that would be available in a regular library. This service is provided by the Library of Congress's National Library Services for the Blind and Physically Handicapped, which owns the special equipment, cassettes, and records, and makes them available to each state through a regional library. A person can obtain, through the state regional library, the special tapes and the cassette player required to play the tapes. Head phones and sound amplifiers are also available. Items are checked out on a loan system, similar to any other library system. Talking Books are recorded on very slow speed and therefore require a special cassette player. An ordinary tape player will not work. Although anyone can purchase audiotapes of books to use in regular tape players, these commercial tapes of books are usually abbreviated and limited in scope; they are not actually "Talking Books" which are provided as special services.

Radio Talking Books is a closed-circuit radio network, accessed by means of a special radio connection; like Talking Books, it is available to those who qualify due to visual or physical impairment. It offers twenty-four-hour, seven-days-per-week programming of best-selling books, magazines, and newspapers, which are read aloud. Contact your regional services office for persons with visual impairment to learn how to obtain this service. Each state has its own title for their state's services. If you are not sure just where to call, contact a librarian, a local rehabilitation office, the activities director at a senior citizens' center, or a therapeutic recreation specialist at a health-care facility in your area for help in finding the right office and the professionals to serve your needs. (See the Related Resources section of this book for contacts that may be useful to you.)

Large-print books, magazines, and newspapers are available through most public libraries. If your local library doesn't have large-print materials on the premises, you can ask about using the interlibrary loan system to help you to get what you want in large print. Large-print computer program formats make it possible to read materials in *very* large print on the computer screen. A computer store is the place to start when you're looking for computers and computer programs adapted to special visual or manual needs. Many bookstores carry audiotapes of books, both abridged and unabridged, as well as audiotapes of old radio programs and other materials.

Offering Choices

Julia

Seventy-year-old Julia was living at the home of her daughter Sandra and Sandra's husband, Brad, following a series of skin graft surgeries after having been in an auto accident. Besides managing Julia's care and following her doctor's instructions, Sandra and Brad planned their strategies for keeping Mom alert and distracted from pain during the weeks she would be with them. They also wanted to be careful not to make Julia any more dependent than necessary.

Sandra wisely made a habit of giving her mother choices rather than simply determining every part of her life for her. "Which of these sheets would you like on your bed this week?" "Coffee or tea for lunch, Mom?" "Raisins in your oatmeal this morning or just plain today?" Sandra knew these were simple choices, but that choices are important. Her mother had been independent until her recent accident, and it would not be good for her to slip into a dependent state of allowing Sandra and Brad to do everything—even make simple choices for her.

Brad's time with Julia usually came when he got home from work at his wallpaper and paint store. Sometimes they played cards or worked together on a crossword puzzle from the day's newspaper. One day at work Brad was about to throw out a series of outdated paint swatches and wallpaper sample books when he decided instead to take them home for Julia to look at. That evening, instead of playing cards, they looked at samples. Brad made a game for them out of opening a page of wallpaper samples and asking Julia questions and discussing her choices. "Which of these do you like best? Which would you use in the living room? In our dining room? In your own kitchen?" Even though her choices weren't going to be put into effect (and both she and Brad knew it), she was actively involved in making choices, discussing her favorites, and reminiscing about wallpaper she had on the walls of her own home. They enjoyed some good conversations as they looked at the designs. Brad was pleased he didn't throw out those sample books.

Sandra gave her mother a chance to keep some control in her life by offering Julia simple choices. You, too, can give the person in your care opportunity to make choices about daily activities such as what to wear, what to eat, what to drink, what activity to do, where to go or not go. When *possible*, make a choice available. Be sure you are ready to accept and act on the choice, however. If you make a choice available, accept the response, whether or not it was the one you wanted. Otherwise, it is better not to make the choice available at all.

Having real choices about even small matters can give a person a greater sense of control over life and help to build self-esteem. Choosing where to place a plant or a picture in the room, whether to open the window or close the drapes, or having a few favorite things in reach can make a difference. When someone feels a sense of personal control, he or she feels more competent and therefore has greater self-esteem, an important point made by J. M. Shary and Seppo Iso-Ahola in their 1989 research. If possible, give the person opportunity to choose and plan activities and then decide when, how long, with whom, and where to do them. That will make the experience free from "have to" and therefore feel more like leisure, which will help to build self-esteem, too.

You can make a game out of simple activity to promote choices that help the use of judgment, identification, recognition, and matching. Brad used the wallpaper books and paint swatches to have discussion with Julia and provide opportunity for her to use her intellectual abilities and make choices. If you are interested in obtaining paint or wallpaper samples, you might request them from a paint and wallpaper store. Sometimes they are willing to give away the outdated samples.

Simplifying Activity

Bert

Bert, thirty-two years old, unmarried, and living alone, recently had a severe car accident that left him with a closed head injury. After coming home from the hospital, Bert received several hours of home care each day, but Harry volunteered to visit twice each week to help keep him mentally alert. Harry found out that Bert had been a news fanatic most of his life. He used to watch news on TV two or three times each day and frequently listened to radio newscasts in his car or workshop. When Harry completed the Checklist of Leisure Favorites with Bert, he discovered Bert still wanted to be in touch with daily news. His attention span was quite short, however, so when Harry read the paper to Bert, he only read the headlines. That seemed to satisfy Bert's need to keep in touch with current events.

Bert's current short attention span and limited interest in outside events led Harry to modify reading the newspaper. Reading whole articles out loud would have been too much for Bert to absorb. You, too, may find it necessary to make modifications and simplify activities to better fit the person in your care. When intellectual activities are either too difficult or too easy in relation to our abilities we dismiss them as "no fun." Through trial and error and close observation of your care receiver's responses, you can plan activities suited to his or her abilities and interests. Notice responses and do only the parts of activities that are comfortable, or change them to suit current abilities. For example, if the person obviously falls asleep while you are reading, you may be reading too long or the material is not interesting. Perhaps the person is not able to understand what you are reading for one reason or another. Or, it could just be that the person is tired. The point is, your observation will tell you to stop reading. However, when you see the person keeps eye contact with you while you read, and listens attentively, perhaps even asking a question about what you are reading, it is clear that the activity is working at this time.

Some intellectual activities have rules or requirements that you can change if you feel the need to. If, for instance, someone enjoys playing games of trivia but thinks slowly now, you might bring up facts from the neighborhood or past life experiences for easy recall, give clues to help, and allow ample time for remembering. You can make up your own rules for games and puzzles. If the person enjoys puzzles but now has limited attention span due to pain or fatigue, try completing most of a puzzle first and then engaging him or her in the final stages of the puzzle or locate a puzzle with fewer pieces. You might find it fun to try word associations. Say the first part and ask for the completion: home sweet—home; nothing ventured—nothing gained; easy come— easy go; there's no place like—home; haste makes—waste. Or say opposites back and forth: hot—cold; sweet—sour; old—young; sun— moon; town—country. Focus on words that are familiar.

Newspapers, magazines, and advertisements are good sources of interesting topics for discussion. Newspapers often have follow-up stories to articles covered in earlier editions. If the person is able to re-member things from day to day, select ongoing current issues to follow according to his or her interests. Ask for opinions. Many magazines print colorful pictures and short articles to look at and read aloud. A good way to use advertising fliers that come through the mail is to draw attention to the ads and their prices. You can share comparative shopping strategies or reminisce about how much similar items used to cost in days gone by. Or, try covering the prices and guessing how much things cost. You both will have some fun with this.

Television and Other Entertainment

Television is a handy, easily available form of entertainment, yet we know very little about its potential for enhancing quality of life among persons receiving care. There is no research to direct us according to what benefits can be derived from viewing particular programs or when and how viewing should be recommended. We do know, how-ever, from the study by Lawton and associates in 1995, that watching television is a common pastime among persons who receive care as well as among the population in general. Therefore, watching televi-sion is a leisure activity that warrants attention here and in future re-search related to care recipients.

Television has many entertaining, educational, and mind-stimulat-ing programs to offer as leisure time activity in the caregiving process. It may be all too convenient, though, to turn on the TV, situate the care receiver in front of the screen, proceed to accomplish other tasks, and pay little attention to what comes on from hour to hour. The person may appear to be engaged in a program simply by virtue of being in the presence of a TV set that is turned on. But sitting before the screen in no way implies mental engagement in a program. Sleeping, day-dreaming, hallucinating, or worrying may be the actual activities tak-ing place; it is difficult to know for sure. The key is to select programs of real interest and promote mental stimulation along with the viewing experience.

Helen

After a slow recovery from hip surgery, Helen's mobility was limited, and she received several hours of home care each week plus volunteer visiting from Miriam, a student nurse. Miriam had only one afternoon each week that fit her schedule for visiting Helen. From the start, Helen informed Miriam that it was okay to come by and visit, but she always spent an hour watching her two favorite soap operas, and if Miriam came at that time, Helen would be busy. Miriam decided to visit immediately following the programs, but she soon found that all Helen wanted to talk about were the characters on her programs, just as though they were neighbors next door. At first Miriam was disheartened by their visits. She had hoped to make a friend of Helen, but all she wanted to talk about were the "soaps."

Finally, Miriam decided to go along with the soap opera idea rather than fight it. So, she rearranged her schedule and came earlier to watch the programs *with* Helen, paying close attention to the characters and the issues involved. When the programs were over, they chatted about the day's episodes and what they expected would happen next. Miriam encouraged discussion about the issues being portrayed on the shows and how they related to current issues in the news and in the community. Sometimes they fantasized about what they would do if they were in those situations. They talked about the characters, who was related to whom, how the families have changed over time, and who were the characters of integrity or evil. They discussed ethical issues like euthanasia, medical costs, sexuality, alcoholism, and drug abuse because they watched those issues evolve on the screen and had plenty to talk about. Miriam and Helen both enjoyed their "soap talk," as they called it, and looked forward to their time together. Miriam's favorite visit turned out to be a little "wedding reception" with cake and tea they shared in front of the TV one afternoon when two characters on the show got married.

Helen loved her soap operas, and Miriam was smart enough to build on the activity that Helen found enjoyable. It is best to use *favorite* programs as the basis of viewing television programs. The Checklist of Favorites will help you find favorite programs, and those are the best shows to schedule as leisure time activity. Rather than simply turning on the set and expecting random programming to be satisfying, be selective about the kind and number of programs. Together, look over a daily or weekly schedule of programs and decide which ones seem to be of interest. That way there is something to look forward to rather than just having the set turned on, letting time go by, hoping the next program will be interesting.

If the person is not mentally able to make program choices or decisions, base program selection on what you know about his or her leisure favorites in general. If the person in your care has cognitive impairment, you may not even be sure whether he or she understands or enjoys the programs. You can make program decisions, however, based on the favorites you know. For someone who enjoyed cooking in the past, cooking programs are a logical choice; for someone who enjoyed gardening, fishing, and the outdoors, programs on those topics seem suitable. Take note of the viewer's responses to programs and find similar programs to the kind that generated an alert response. In his 1995 book *Keeping Busy: A Handbook of Activities for Persons with Dementia*, activities specialist James R. Dowling suggests that the best programs for persons with dementia tend to be reruns of the "Golden Oldies" such as "I Love Lucy," "Ozzie and Harriet," and the shows of Jack Benny, George Burns, and other entertainers from that era.

Not only can TV programs be used for entertainment, they are good for mental stimulation. In the case of Helen, we see that Miriam used their discussion time as opportunity to activate Helen's mind about the characters, their family histories, and ethical and current issues, and guess what might happen next, and what she would do if she were in the same situations. Therapeutic recreation educator Annette Logan explained in 1985 that soap operas lend themselves to mentally stimulating discussions, and people who follow the programs can be helped to connect characters, events, and issues. Discussing television programs before and after the viewing is useful and mentally stimulating beyond the actual program time. Not every program must be discussed, however, in order to be beneficial or entertaining. What's most important is for the individual to be engaged in a program rather than sitting mentally "numb" in front of noise coming from the TV set hour after hour.

Videocassette tapes can also provide mental stimulation and entertainment if you have a videocassette recorder. Besides renting videos from commercial stores, you can obtain videos from many libraries which carry videocassettes on various topics of interest. Generally, they can be checked out just like books. Contact your librarian for information about specific titles and topics available in your area. If you have a college or university nearby, the library and various academic departments may also have videos available for your use.

Reminiscence

Recreational reminiscence is an activity that keeps the mind active and is also pleasurable. People of all ages find enjoyment in relating stories about past events. Reminiscing allows an individual to tell unique stories that are important in the life experience. In their 1990 book *Reminiscing Together: Ways to Help Us Keep Mentally Fit As We Grow Older*, Howard Thorsheim and Bruce Roberts relate reminiscing to bringing out souvenirs of the past: "Our unique experiences are like precious pictures or other mementos stored in a treasure box. We bring them out from time to time to admire them and the experiences they remind us of. The more we take them out, the more familiar and dear they become to us. If, however, we keep them in their box most of the time, we almost forget that we have them" (p. 5).

Here are a few helpful hints about how to bring out those treasures from the memory, and "prime the pump" for stories. Rather than simply asking your care receiver to recall an event or meaningful memory, you will have more success if you present an actual object to "trigger" the memory. For example, if you say, "Grandma, tell me about your wedding day," she will have to scan the files of her mind to recall something from that event. She may feel "on the spot" if she can't think of something quickly. But if you show her a photo taken on her wedding day and with it say, "Grandma, tell me about the wedding dress you wore in this picture," she will be able to recognize herself and the situation. She will find it easier to tell a story to go with it because the photo prompts her recognition rather than requiring her simply to recall the event. In her extensive writing about reminiscence, professor of therapeutic recreation at the University of Minnesota Caroline Weiss suggested that providing a prop expedites retrieving information from memory through recognition rather than recall. We can see what this means in the following case of Luis.

Luis

Ted, an in-home health aide, worked part time as caregiver to Luis, aged thirty-eight, who was approaching late stages of AIDS. Ted discovered that Luis enjoyed thinking about his high school and college days. This gave Ted ideas about reminiscing that could be useful in diverting Luis's attention from pain, and keeping him interested in life. As Ted looked around Luis's house for things he might use to activate Luis's memory, he noticed a drawer labeled "maps" and asked Luis if they could look at them together. To Ted's surprise, Luis seemed eager to bring them out. The maps were marked with evidence of plans and routes of Luis's earlier trips with college buddies.

When Ted had time apart from other caregiving duties, he took one map at a time and asked Luis to tell stories about where he and his buddies had been, where they stopped, what they did in special places. Luis pointed out a shelf where Ted found two photo albums that he could use to fit into Luis's stories. In spite of pain and fatigue, Luis communicated through the maps and pictures, tracing routes with his fingers and matching pictures to the maps. One afternoon, while they looked at a map of Yellowstone National Park, Ted got paper and pencil and asked Luis to draw a map of Old Faithful. The site seemed to be clear in his mind. He drew a winding road that led to a number of smoking geysers and the massive eruption of Old Faithful. Ted easily "got the picture," and they had a lively discussion about the smell of sulfur at Old Faithful. Luis didn't need to tell long stories in order to be mentally involved. Both found that time flew when they reminisced like this, and Luis stuck with the activity for several minutes each time, in spite of his short attention span.

Since Luis enjoyed many trips with college buddies, the maps of those trips moved his memory to remember the good times. Many other objects can do the same thing. To activate memories when reminiscing, use actual objects such as maps, photos, household items, music, scrapbooks, newspaper clippings, antiques, foods, spices, recipe books, seed catalogs, magazine pictures, posters, pets, invitations received for past events, greeting cards, holiday decorations, items of clothing, tools, seeds, fruits, vegetables, toys, jewelry, and on and on the list can go. Remember, reminiscing will come easier and be more specific if you use props in your conversation. As Caroline Weiss has pointed out, *actual objects* provide a bridge to the circumstances in which the memories first registered. Holding a pair of suspenders and yanking at the straps is likely to prompt a story about someone who wore suspenders; holding and smelling a small cedar box will take the memory back to a time and place where there is a story. Have some fun finding props to "trigger" the memory and enjoy the stories that unfold.

Because maps are familiar items in most people's lives, they are readily available and easily used in reminiscence. A friend of mine carries maps of Minnesota and surrounding states when he visits a friend in a nursing home who likes to talk about places she lived and visited. She enjoys showing him the exact routes and locations that were part of her life; and they have lively visits. In 1987, Weiss developed an interesting activity which she called "mapping" and suggested a variety of ideas about how to use maps to stimulate a connection to a person's past. Some of her suggestions include (a) drawing maps about the "growing up" years: maps of favorite rooms in the house—the kitchen, the living room—maps showing where the furniture was placed, who used this room, what went on there; a map of the backyard, the farm, the garden, the city, the old neighborhood, the old school; (b) drawing maps of places visited on trips and vacations, the landscapes, monuments, special attractions, significant memories; (c) making original maps such as cutting and arranging pictures from a seed catalog to map out a flower garden, or illustrating dance steps with paper footprints. A person does not need to be an accomplished artist to map out important memories and tell related meaningful stories. Often a map calls forth memories of feelings, sounds, and aromas associated with a particular place. Have some fun with maps!

Reminiscing can be recreational, pleasurable, and meaningful, a point made in 1991 by gerontologist Edmund Sherman. In caregiving you will want to pursue memories and stories for their *recreational* value, not for therapeutic purposes. Many experts recommend that *therapeutic reminiscence* be left to qualified psychotherapists who can help people to relive *and resolve* old conflicts. *Recreational reminiscing*, on the other hand, is pleasurable and has benefits for both storyteller and listener. The storyteller has opportunity for reviewing accomplishments, realizing past and present competencies, and enjoying comforting feelings from the past; benefits for the listener include a legacy of wisdom, historical and cultural information, and a better relationship with the storyteller. Recreational reminiscence is an ideal leisure activity to build the "us" between caregiver and care receiver.

Telling life stories will, however, bring up both happy and sad times, laughter and tears, and a wide variety of feelings. Let them all come out. No need to fear a few tears any more than hearty laughter. Tears may stem from extreme joy or pride, sadness or regret. Try to be comfortable with all the emotions. Listen and be reassuring rather than try to fix the story or its outcome. You can acknowledge and validate feelings to let a person know those feelings are important, a method supported by validation specialist Naomi Feil and by Caroline Weiss. Validating a feeling means to acknowledge it and accept that the person has that feeling. You might validate a sad feeling with a comment such as, "Yes, that must have been a difficult time in your life" or acknowledge anger by saying, "Oh, I can see why you felt that way." In recreational reminiscence, it may be wise to validate a feeling and then move on to another subject. If a story seems too painful to pursue, it may be helpful to leave that topic and go on to another. If an upsetting topic with unresolved issues keeps recurring, consult a professional for guidance.

In their book *Guiding Autobiography Groups for Older Adults: Exploring the Fabric of Life*, gerontologists James E. Birren and Donna E. Deutchman suggest that tears not be taken too seriously in the midst of reminiscing: "It is not a sign something has gone wrong. It is a sign something is going right." But they suggest that once the tears begin to flow, you must decide when it is time to move on. Simple nonverbal cues such as a smile, a quick hug, a pat on the hand, or the passing of a box of tissues may send a message of empathy while letting the person know that it is time to move along.

Pay close attention to the stories that come up. Take the role of an active listener. Use good eye contact and give "interested" responses. Take time to listen as though you have heard the story for the first time, even if you've heard the same story many times before. Try not to engage in other activity such as folding laundry or cleaning the house while reminiscing. Let the storytelling occupy your time and interest. Use open-ended questions if the storyteller is able to respond; closed-ended questions will be more appropriate for a person who is withdrawn. Open-ended questions leave room for a variety of responses yet give direction to the information you are seeking. These are examples of open-ended questions: "What were the people like when you traveled through Alaska?" "What was your country school like?" "What were the house parties like in those days?" "What did you think of the big city when you first moved there?" Closed-ended questions, on the other hand, invite specific answers: "Were the roads paved when you traveled through Alaska?" "How many grades were in one room in your country school?" "Did you meet Dad at a house party?" "Were you excited when you first went to the big city?" You may find both kinds of questions useful, but the withdrawn person will find it easier to respond to the closed-ended questions. Because it is sometimes difficult to determine whether or not a person is withdrawn, you might begin with open-ended questions. If you are not getting a response, switch to closed-ended questions in order to draw more simplified answers to your questions. Your attentive listening and interactive responses will help to build your relationship with the storyteller. You may also enjoy compiling some lasting evidence of your shared reminiscence. Celia's story below will give you some ideas.

Celia

After being diagnosed with slowly progressing cancer, Celia, eighty-seven, lived with her daughter Kay and son-in-law Bob, who provided the supervision she needed, mostly during evening and nighttime hours. Because they knew her well, they knew Celia had a variety of interests, but most of all she loved to tell stories about her life. She had kept diaries for years and also had notebooks filled with accounts of trips she had taken with her husband and family over her lifetime. Kay realized her mother held a wealth of family history that soon could be lost. She and Bob thought it would be fun to help Celia preserve her knowledge and stories to pass on to her family. Celia agreed.

During some of their evening time together, Kay and Bob engaged Celia in conversation about events of her life. With Celia's consent, Bob made audiotapes of their conversations. He kept the sessions short so Celia didn't become overtired. Because Kay was familiar with many of her mom's stories, she could guide the conversation to include various eras of her life such as: growing up on the farm; school days; courtship and marriage; children and grandchildren.

Later, Kay typed some of the stories onto the computer and printed them so Celia could see her words in print. She was quite pleased about her work and amazed that Kay and Bob were so interested. When Kay suggested making a little book out of the stories and giving it to the children and grandchildren for Christmas, Celia glowed and agreed.

They worked together to find important newspaper clippings and photos to include. It turned out to be a modest little book duplicated at a copy shop and bound with plastic loops. Celia entitled it: *My Days Gone By*. In it were stories about hard winters on the farm, how her dad raised horses, how her parents couldn't afford to send her to high school, when she met her husband, how she coped with illnesses of her children, and how proud she was of her family. When Christmas rolled around, her children and grandchildren were thrilled to receive a copy of her book and told Celia it was the best present she could ever give them.

When Celia's book turned out to be such a "hit" in the family, Bob decided to go one step further and capture Celia on videotape, telling more of her stories. She agreed to just sit and talk with Kay while Bob made the tape. Kay asked her questions that led to stories that made them both laugh and cry. In just thirty minutes, they secured more of Celia's life stories in another valuable family treasure.

Perhaps the way you record a few memories will not be as elaborate as Celia's book or a videotape, but do what you can to capture memories for years to come. It can be stimulating and fun to reminisce and preserve memories in a tangible form. Lasting evidence provides opportunity to pass on a legacy of memories to family and other people who may be interested. The format may be simple or sophisticated depending on interest and available resources. These are some possible ways to preserve memories: audiotapes, videotapes, books, computer-printed booklets, letters, scrapbooks, diaries, recipe books, photo albums, journals, posters, wall hangings, collages. Memories can be expressed in poetry, drawings, music, and original songs. You can enjoy the *process* of producing the document as well as the final product. Then, reviewing the product brings ongoing leisure experience each time you bring it out to look at or talk about. With so many pleasurable features, it is no wonder reminiscing is a favorite leisure activity among people of all ages.

Keeping the Senses Stimulated

All information comes to us through our senses. Everything we ever learned came to us through our senses—our sense of sight, hearing, taste, smell, and touch. Therefore, if we are to help others stay alert, we need to keep feeding them information through their senses.

Hazel

Tom was the family member designated to visit his grandmother, Hazel, during afternoon hours. Hazel had been diagnosed with dementia a year ago. She also had limited vision. Now, she needed supervision most of the time. She slept very little during the day hours, so Tom figured some activities would help her during the afternoon visits. Because of Hazel's dementia, their conversations were limited. She seemed to have no interest in watching TV. Tom found, though, that she was able to respond to things for at least short periods of time, especially if he went slowly, one thing at a time. Tom had learned that stimulation of the senses is especially important for people who are withdrawn or who may have some degree of dementia. So, Tom decided to find activities that help to stimulate the senses.

Sense of smell. The kitchen was a perfect place to start. The spice cupboard was a natural. Hazel had always been a good cook, she was familiar with spices, and the smells would be a good way to keep her sense of smell more keen. Tom brought Hazel to the table and gave her one spice bottle at a time. They took a good whiff of each open bottle—first Hazel, then Tom—and he watched her reaction. Some aromas, such as the cinnamon, vanilla flavoring, maple flavoring, cloves, made her smile; others, such as dried onions, Tabasco sauce, garlic, made her face pinch. They laughed over some and sneezed after the pepper. Tom liked this activity; he decided to do it often. On other days, Tom brought scented hand lotion, which he gave Hazel to rub into her hands. Sometimes he brought perfume, potpourri, scented candles, and scented soaps for Hazel to smell and enjoy.

Sense of hearing. One idea led to another. Sounds, Tom thought. Oh, yes, he could find sounds that would help Hazel stay alert, too. He gathered several bells, a music box, two windup toys, wind chimes, and his tape recorder with a variety of music. Listening to a few sounds was an activity Tom could count on lasting a good ten minutes. He was pleased to get Hazel's attention for that long. Sometimes he played soothing music; it seemed to calm her. She seemed to like it, and sometimes she moved her hands as though she were directing the orchestra.

Sense of touch. Tom put several items in what he called the "feely bag" (actually a pillow case), which was his hiding place for the textured objects that he used to get Hazel's attention and help keep her sense of touch alert. In his "feely bag" he had such things as a bumpy gourd, a toothbrush, an emery board, a silver dollar, a wooden doll, a large ball of cotton, a rubber ball, a crushed paper napkin, and a plastic box. He was careful to include items that were safe and in no way could harm Hazel. After a few times, when he brought out his "feely bag" Hazel immediately smiled and reached in for something. She seemed to enjoy the textures. Sometime Tom wet a cloth with warm water to use as a napkin after meals. Hazel willingly wiped her face and hands while enjoying the pleasurable warmth. He decided to warm her towels from time to time.

Sense of taste. When Tom visited, he tried to add zest to their snacks. He did things like vary the flavor of tea he served Hazel, spread different kinds of jam on their crackers, sliced fruit and gave Hazel one slice at a time so she could enjoy each bite, and included crunchy vegetables when possible. Once in a while they shared a bowl of popcorn.

Sense of sight. Because Hazel's vision was limited, Tom had a great challenge keeping her visually stimulated. He knew bright colors and large print were important. He also knew contrasting colors, such as black print on yellow paper, are easier to see. He brought in things like brightly colored balloons, colored paper napkins, large bright flowers—sometimes real, sometimes made of silk. He found his time with Hazel more interesting for him, too, when they did activities together that stimulated their senses.

Tom was successful in bringing sensory stimulation into a wide range of daily living activities. It may take some thinking and effort on your part, but you, too, can use daily opportunities to promote sensory stimulation for the person in your care. Occasionally Tom set up specific activity time to bring out things for Hazel to touch, smell, taste, see, and hear. There are many opportunities throughout the day for keeping senses alert. Let the person being cared for help with doing dishes, maybe just to get hands in the sudsy water. Give him or her a fluffy pillow to stroke while sitting on the sofa. Think of things like folding towels, smelling flowers, putting on perfume and enjoying the fragrance, handling an apple before it is washed and prepared for eating, or feeling the edges of a comb before using it. Be creative. Look around and see what there is to be touched, smelled, tasted, seen, and heard in everyday living.

For people who are "difficult to reach" due to physical, emotional, or mental disability or because of pain, fatigue, or dementia, sensory stimulation serves as a nonverbal "connecting bridge" and may be one of the few successful means of relating to them. Because the sense of touch, through the skin, is the largest sense, use touch especially when all else fails. Here are a few ideas: a warm, gentle manicure complete with nail polish (if suitable); warm towels after a bath or while resting; hand and arm massage with warm lotion; a cool cloth on the forehead; a warm, gentle foot and leg rub; a warm, gentle back and shoulder rub; a sincere hug; a gentle kiss on the cheek; fresh bed sheets; a soft, favorite pillow; a plush stuffed animal; a cuddly real animal. Use a variety of the ideas discussed above and in the summary as your tools to "reach" someone. Use especially strong scents and fragrances, brightly colored objects, pleasant sounds, and memorable tastes. For instance, you are likely to get some response from the person smelling lilacs, looking at bright rainbow fabric, feeling silky material, or tasting ice cream or sliced oranges, because of the intensity of the stimulation. Everyone is different, though, and you cannot predict the exact type or length of response you will get, so try several things. Stimulate *all* the senses and you will be more likely to make "connections" with the person.

For some persons, especially those who have dementia, it may be important to avoid using many stimulating things at the same time. Too many things going on at once can cause what is called a "sensory overload," a condition that simply means too much stimulation to the senses at the same time. When that happens for some people, they become more confused, agitated, and unable to focus on any one thing. To prevent sensory overload while you do an activity, avoid competing noises in the room such as background music on the radio, and avoid distracting movements from hanging decorations or other people coming and going. It will be important to enjoy just one thing at a time. Listen to the sound of a bell or feel silky fabric—one at a time. Do not rush. *Take time* with each item to make the most of the experience, yet avoid the frustration of too much at once.

In their book *Working with Older Adults: Group Process and Techniques*, Irene Burnside and Mary Gwynne Schmidt address the issue of safety when working with persons who have cognitive impairment. As a caregiver, when you minimize the danger of your care recipient's experiencing harm, you increase the person's independence, because he or she can freely participate in activity. Among the helpful hints offered by Burnside and Schmidt are the following, which are especially useful when using sensory stimulation with a person who has dementia. (1) Avoid artificial fruits, etc. that look like they can be eaten; the person may not be able to detect the difference between the artificial item and the real thing and may try to eat it. (2) Be careful with hot tea or coffee as well as very cold items. (3) Do not put refreshments in view until you are ready to serve them; the person may eat them immediately, not realizing there is a set time for eating. (4) Avoid jingling keys as a visual or auditory stimulation; keys may be a cue to get up and go someplace when that is not the case. (5) If you keep things in plastic bags, keep the bags out of the person's reach.

Sensory stimulation has the added feature of triggering the memory for reminiscence. For instance, a plush animal may not only be soft and comforting to hold but may be a source of conversation as well, as noted by nursing professor Gloria Francis and doctoral candidate Anita Baly in their 1986 report on the effects of plush animals on older adults in nursing homes. Keen memories are often associated with sense stimulators such as smooth, varnished wood, rough stucco, sand, a furry kitten, a hug, alfalfa, fried chicken, cedar, smoke, and mothballs, onions, turpentine, diesel fuel, dill pickles. When you combine those ideas and all the ideas in this chapter into leisure moments, you are bound to rouse memories that bring up fabulous life stories. Enjoy them all!

Summary

A wide variety of leisure activities help to keep the mind active and provide enjoyment besides. Even while receiving care, most people still continue to enjoy mental activity. Educational opportunities are available through options such as classes, television, videotapes, books, newspapers, magazines, mental games, and sensory stimulation activities. Recreational reminiscence not only keeps the mind active but creates a communication bridge between care receiver and caregiver.

Ideas for Intellectual Activities

cut out coupons

do crossword puzzles

learn a language

listen to a talk show

look at magazines

make a scrapbook

play cards

play dice games

put together puzzles

read newspapers

read stories out loud

solve riddles

teach someone a skill

tell stories

write in a journal

write poetry

other _____

discuss current events

learn card tricks

learn magic tricks

listen to Talking Books

look at old photos

organize cupboards

play checkers, chess

play mystery games

read books

read poetry

reminisce

solve word problems

tell jokes

write a grocery list

write letters

write a story

_____

Ideas for Reminiscing

To activate memories in recreational reminiscence, use actual objects such as:

antiques

books

dishes

fashions

fruits

grocery ads or coupons

jewelry

lumber

maps

photos

poetry

quilts

seeds

baked goods

comic books

farm magazines

flowers and weeds

greeting cards

invitations

knickknacks

magazines

music books

plaques, trophies, certificates

newspaper clippings

scrapbooks

seed catalogs

sewing supplies	school lunch bucket
stones, rocks, sea shells	tools
toys	videotapes
vegetables	other _____

Ideas for Sensory Stimulation

Sense of smell: aromas, such as:

apple sauce	aromatic tea
catnip	cedar
cinnamon	cloves
cocoa	coffee
dried onions	garlic
herbs	incense
Italian seasoning	ketchup
lemon juice	maple flavoring
mustard	peanut butter
perfume	pickles
potpourri	roses
sawdust	scented candle
scented lotion	scented soap
sea weed	spaghetti sauce
Tabasco sauce	tanning lotion
vanilla flavoring	wildflowers
other _____	_____

Sense of hearing: sounds, such as:

audiotapes	barking dog
bells	bird calls
coins	cuckoo clock
drums	grandfather clock
harmonica	humming
music box	ocean sounds
piano	plastic cartons
pots and pans	purring, meowing cat
reading aloud	soothing music
traffic	typewriter

wind chimes   windup toys

other _____   _____

Sense of touch—textured objects and things to feel such as:

acorns   bubbles
bumpy gourd   comb
cool cloth on forehead   emery board
foot rub   gently blowing fan
hand massage with lotion   jar rings, lids
large ball of cotton   makeup
manicure   marbles
nylon stockings   opening a zipper
outdoor breeze   paper flowers
pedicure   pin cushion
pinecones   plastic egg
plush stuffed animal   polished stones
pottery   potting soil
pulling elastic   ribbons
rocking chair   rubber ball
rubber bands   silver dollar
spray of a water fountain   toothbrush
toys   warm towel
other _____   _____

Sense of taste—variety of tastes, such as:

applesauce   berries
cheese   cookie dough
cotton candy   crackers
dessert toppings   flavored coffee
flavored tea   honey
hot chocolate   ice cream
jams and jellies   ketchup
lemonade   marshmallows
mustard   peanut butter
pickles   pineapple
popcorn   pudding
salad dressings   sliced fruit

snow cones	soda pop
variety of juices	various nuts
vegetables	watermelon
other _____	_____

Sense of sight—bright and colored items such as:

aquarium with fish	art reproductions
brightly colored balloons	brightly colored paper napkins
catalogs	color wheel of paint samples
colorful posters	computer games
floral print fabric	kaleidoscope
large, bright flowers	large, colorful decorations
large-leafed plants	large-print written material
magazine pictures	mobiles
shiny jewelry	terrarium
wallpaper samples	other _____

CHAPTER FIVE

Emotional and Expressive Activity

BENEFITS
Emotional activities give one opportunity for a variety of expressions and moods. They help us to express feelings and individuality, increase self-esteem, take risks, feel consequences, have fun.

The freedom that we associate with leisure includes freedom to be ourselves and to express ourselves freely. The activities that fit into the emotional and expressive domain bring out the individuality of a person and offer opportunities for a great deal of fun. A wide variety of activities help us do that. In this chapter you will find discussion of the following:

☆ The importance of humor in the caregiving process
☆ Building self-esteem through leisure experiences
☆ Opportunities for self-expression in leisure time
☆ Hobbies and service projects

Enjoying the Magic of Humor

Laughter can supply a certain magic that helps people get through hard times. It can be very useful in a caregiving situation, but we need to be sure the humor we use is appropriate to the person and situation. Not everyone is in a "think funny" frame of mind at all times, especially when in need of care or when dealing with pain and illness. It will be important for you to know your care receiver well, and understand the kind of humor that is suitable to the person and the situation. The best kind of humor seems to be the kind where we can laugh at ourselves and then laugh with others over silly, everyday things that happen. I like the little saying that says, "Laugh at yourself, and the world laughs *with* you; laugh *at* others, and you laugh alone."

In the preface to his 1995 book *The Magic of Humor in Caregiving*, educational psychologist James R. Sherman suggests that if you can find something to laugh at, no matter how serious your situation, you'll see caregiving in a new and refreshing way. "That doesn't mean you're being disrespectful of your care receiver or the condition that brings you together," Sherman writes. "Nor does it mean that you have to find humor in everything. It just means you've tried to lighten the impact of one of life's misfortunes and tried to make your situation more enjoyable."

Just because a person is ill or disabled, in need of care and supervision, or living under less than ideal circumstances doesn't mean all the moments must be heavy. You can be on the lookout for ways to bring chuckles into the day. You can use humor as a means of relaxing and coping, too. Therapeutic recreation educators Francis A. McGuire and Rosangela Boyd pointed out in 1993 that humor has both a preventive and a maintenance function. They summarized studies that show humor has a positive influence on physical and mental health and enables people to face their fears. Laughter doesn't just feel good, it also causes deep, relaxed breathing and for a short time clears the mind of all thoughts and emotions except what's causing the laughter. Physician Bernie Siegel explained in 1986 that physiologists have found that muscle relaxation and anxiety cannot exist together, and that the relaxation response following a good laugh lasts up to forty-five minutes. What's more, laughter begets laughter. Hopefully we have all felt the momentum of "getting the giggles"—one laugh building on another, until finally we couldn't stop. Very likely, when it was all over, the relaxation response left us feeling better than before.

You don't need to be a stand-up comedian to enjoy humor, laugh, and reap the benefits. In fact, most of us don't do very well when it comes to telling jokes. You don't need to. Daily activities bring up silly circumstances—that is, if we have the mind-set to see them as funny. When we "think funny" about daily events, they go better. I agree with Bernie Siegel, who says that one of the best measures of mental health is the ability to laugh at oneself in a gently mocking way. Depending on our frame of mind, we can feel irritation or have a chuckle over routine occurrences such as dropping silverware, burning the toast, or misbuttoning a shirt. In her 1992 book *Taking Care of Me: How Caregivers Can Effectively Deal with Stress*, Katherine L. Karr wrote that humor is an attitude, a state of mind, a way of placing in perspective events life hands us. A humorous interpretation of an unsettling event can go a long way in breaking its hold on us. I remember my father's reaction years ago when one of his friends teased him after noticing Dad had on one black sock and one brown sock. "Oh yes," Dad joked, "and I have another pair just like it at home!" He was clever to laugh at himself and enjoy the moment.

Goldie

Since Chester retired, he spent most of his days caring for his wife, Goldie, whose multiple sclerosis had progressed to the point where she needed assistance with most of her activities of daily living. Chester learned early in this arrangement that they had better continue to laugh a lot, just as they always had, or this situation would be impossible for them both. Chester tried to keep a lighthearted frame of mind and do what he could to keep their spirits up.

When the newspaper arrived every morning, Chester pulled out the comic strip section before reading anything else, just as he had done in their early years. He shared with Goldie their dose of comics before breakfast. When the mail arrived, the chances of getting a chuckle were quite good, since Chester had enlisted the help of their four children, the in-laws, and five grandchildren to keep up their supply of comics and clever quotes. When "the kids" had asked Chester how they could be of help to him, he had suggested they might send in the mail some humorous items from time to time. Luckily, they were good about following through on this request as often as they could, and mail time was a much anticipated time of the day. Goldie liked to have the most humorous items stuck on the refrigerator with magnets, although she often kidded that they would be seen more often if they were taped to the *inside* of the refrigerator.

Chester also designated a small table at the entrance of their bedroom as the "humor spot" in the house. Here he placed little surprises from time to time and watched to see how long it would take before

Goldie found them. He would do things like cut out silly or colorful pictures from magazines and add them to the "humor spot." Sometimes, when he went downtown, he'd pick up a windup toy from the children's section of a store and slip it onto the table when he got home. He'd wait for Goldie to find it and ask for help to get it going. He loved to see them giggle over such simple things. He knew that a friend of theirs thought they acted like children, but he had always claimed that kids didn't have a monopoly on toys and fun. Besides, the youngest grandchildren were always eager to stop by and play with grandpa and grandma's "toys."

The children and grandchildren had given them a VCR for Christmas, and since then they rented two or three videos per week. Chester checked with Goldie about her preferences for the week, and she often selected a comedy film. Since Goldie didn't get out of the house very often, the videos helped keep both of them in touch with current movies, and the comedies kept them laughing.

That "think funny" mind-set we see in Chester helped Goldie and him cope with their daily living. If you can feel comfortable using humor along the way, there are a variety of techniques that can be useful: be willing to laugh at yourself and say silly things about what happens in daily life; read the comic strip section of the newspaper; use comical expressions and quips; tape humorous items on the refrigerator; rent a comedy video and watch it together. Encourage laughing out loud, not only smiles and quiet chuckles. Use the Checklist of Leisure Favorites to find favorite humorous items.

Both you and the person in your care can have some fun if you read out loud some humor sections from an issue of the *Reader's Digest* or other sources. Reading humorous stories out loud will give you a chance to laugh together. If your selections are short they won't demand deep attention and you will be able to laugh at punch lines often. Let the stories you read lead you to your own funny stories to share and enjoy.

Be sure to select humorous reading materials yourself in your own reading time as well. If there are other family members with you in your caregiving situation, enjoy reading humorous items out loud and enjoy other silliness among yourselves. Let yourselves enjoy hearty laughter as a wonderful physical and emotional stress releaser.

Like Goldie and Chester, you might want to designate a place in the house as the "humor spot." Here, place little humorous surprises from time to time and watch to see how long it takes for someone to find them. If your care receiver does not leave his or her bed or room, set up the humor spot at the bedside or in the room; select items to look at and enjoy together. Items might include silly or colorful pictures from magazines, windup toys, cute plaques, a music box, jack-in-the-box, bubble machine, photos, quotes, stuffed animals, and knickknacks you think will bring a smile. Or, perhaps the "humor spot" is the ceiling, above the bed, in view during waking hours, where posters and other decorations or mobiles can provide entertainment.

If this idea fits your caregiving situation, ask family members or friends to send quips, quotes, and jokes in the mail; this adds a chuckle to opening the mail and gives you both something to look forward to.

If you collect or tell jokes, riddles, word quizzes, and silly word games, you can have a few laughs both at the time you find them and again when you share them with the person being cared for. Just a word of caution, however, about jokes. It may be helpful to screen jokes before bringing them to your care receiver to eliminate any that might be offensive to the person. As you get to know someone better, you will get to know his or her favorite kinds of humor, which will make your selections easier.

Influencing Self-Esteem and Mood

It is not news to you, if you are a caregiver, that illness and disability create twists and turns in life that weren't there before. Some of these changes have to do with schedule, routines, or even how to best place the furniture in the house. But some of the changes are taking place in the person who is in need of care. He or she may become more sensitive to loud sounds, for example, or, ultimately, may not be able to hear as well as formerly. Here are some other ways in which the person in your care may be changing:

⇨ difference in perception (in how things look, sound, smell, feel, or taste)
⇨ changes in judgment and ability to reason
⇨ changes in ability to pay attention

⇨ a different sense of one's own body (how the body looks and feels)

⇨ changes in what feels hot or cold

⇨ changes in how long it takes to complete even simple tasks

⇨ sense of touch may be less keen

⇨ taste and smell may be less keen

⇨ eye sight may be less sharp

⇨ changes in perception of light (whether dim or bright)

⇨ changes in what sounds loud or soft

⇨ moods may vary from week to week, day to day, or more often

Sometimes these changes have a negative impact on how a person feels about himself or herself. Part of your job, then, is to do what you can to build self-esteem in spite of ongoing changes.

Florence

Florence, a sixty-eight-year-old grandmother, showed signs of early dementia. Family members were concerned about how long she could live by herself. So far, she had been receiving several hours of home care each week, but it seemed she soon would need ongoing care.

One Sunday afternoon when her granddaughter Jeannette visited, she noticed Florence had not combed her hair that day, and very likely not for a few days. Jeannette told her grandmother that she had a little time this afternoon and asked if she would like a "make over." They both laughed, and Jeannette promised she was good at it. Florence thought it would be fun. Jeannette was sure it would help her grandmother feel better. They began with a hair wash.

When they got to the bathroom, Florence looked in the mirror and began to cry. She did not look like her well-kept self, and seemed to realize the consequences of her deteriorating condition. Very wisely, Jeannette distracted her grandmother from the mirror, began washing her hair, took time to set it and blow-dry it. Then she spent time combing out Florence's hair in her favorite style. When they were finished, Jeannette gave the mirror to her grandmother, and again, to Jeannette's surprise, she began to cry. Jeannette didn't know what to do. She thought she had done a great job of the "make over," but Grandma still wasn't satisfied. Rather than dwelling on it, Jeannette suggested they have a snack, and they finished their visit with some cookies and iced tea.

That week, Jeannette asked some questions of a friend who works at a long-term care facility. The friend told Jeannette that sometimes a person's perception of self changes with dementia. Perhaps what Florence saw in the mirror was not exactly what Jeannette or other people were seeing. The friend told Jeannette about several strategies the family might try to help Florence feel better about herself. One thing they could do was cover the mirrors with pictures or wallpaper so Florence would not have to concern herself with her changing looks. They might also help Grandmother keep up her grooming so she would feel her best at all times.

Florence provides just one example of how complicated the changes in perception can be when dementia, illness, or disability set in. Do what you can to make the activities of daily living into moments of pleasure that promote looking and feeling good. Body image and body awareness can strongly influence how a person feels about himself or herself. Taking time to comb hair, put on a light coating of lipstick, wash and polish fingernails, put on a favorite shirt, and enjoy the view in the mirror are important activities that bring simple joys and build self-esteem. Try placing a comfortably warm or cool cloth on the forehead, massaging hands or feet with lotion, gently brushing hair with a soft brush, giving a manicure or a foot rub.

Try to help the person receiving care to continue doing tasks of daily living, grooming, and hygiene so he or she can feel as good as possible. Use strategies like covering mirrors if that helps. On the other hand, looking in the mirror may help the person make adjustments to the new self. When your care receiver's condition brings continuing physical changes, as in the case of progressive disease, there often are accompanying emotional changes that influence self-esteem. Remember, you want the person to feel good about himself or herself through all the activities you do. Building self-esteem is a basic purpose behind the leisure experiences you share with the person in your care. Some of those experiences include basic care activities because they can produce the good feelings we associate with leisure.

Also, as the provider of care, it will be to your advantage to look after your own appearance too. You don't need to attend tanning sessions at a salon or spend money on new hairdos to keep up your self-image. Just be comfortable with yourself so you can enjoy life as much as possible. The idea is to feel good about yourself just as you want the other person to feel good. For some of us, we feel better when we are comfortable about how we look. Take enough time for your self-care activities, such as bathing, dressing, and primping, so you can enjoy them and feel good about your appearance.

Tina

Eight-year-old Tina was confined to a body cast for twelve weeks due to hip surgery. When Tina returned home from the hospital to complete her recovery, her mother, Dorothy, assumed the caregiver role and quickly realized the challenge ahead. Tina was a normal child with high energy and varied interests, but her moods seemed to be in high swing every day. She was demanding and cried easily, more from frustration than from pain, it seemed. She could giggle with a video, then quickly scowl at her mother at meal time. What to do? Would the family just have to put up with these moods for the duration of her confinement? Dorothy invited Tina's friends over for activities from time to time, which helped, but was not the solution they needed.

One morning, her mother declared, "Today is backwards day, Anit!" Tina finally figured it out—"Anit" was her name—backwards. Her mother brought a hamburger to her for breakfast and walked backwards into the room with her sweatshirt back in front. Tina giggled and tried to figure out how to say some words backwards. The idea kept her guessing—what would Mom do next? Lunch brought meat loaf and upside-down cake; the cake had to be eaten first; no complaints from Tina. Of course, cereal and toast were on the "breakfast" menu for supper. Her brother Kurt (today called "Truk") got into the act too, trying to put together a puzzle with Tina—picture side down, of course. Tina and her mother giggled a great deal that day, acting silly, trying to figure out how to do things backwards.

Mood swings can be common during times of illness and disability. You will want to pay attention to mood swings, because they may indicate changes in physical or psychological condition. If you have any concerns about the cause or extent of the mood changes, it's a good idea to get a professional opinion—perhaps from the person's doctor. Sometimes a bad mood persists and the person does not feel like engaging in humorous escapades. When that is the situation, be wise enough to "back off" until a better moment arises.

It is possible, though, that simple "fun" activities can help to stabilize, or at least change, a person's mood, and both you and the other person can share something that "breaks the spell" of a bad mood. Focus on activities that produce fun and laughter. Even short periods of mood stability count. Tina's mother knew that she would face the challenge of Tina's moods again tomorrow, but for this one day, "backwards day" helped, and everyone in the household felt better, at least long enough to regain some energy and peace of mind.

Other humorous "mood changers" include using puppets as playful characters who carry a message or who can be used as partners in dramatic, self-expressive play; dressing up in costumes for special occasions or just for fun; wearing a silly hat; telling "let's pretend" stories; blowing bubbles; reading aloud stories of exaggerated characters—animals that talk, or gentle giants; learning magic tricks and then performing them for others; drawing cartoons; playing with windup toys and interactive toys; and clowning. Many of these suggestions are offered by nursing professor Ann H. Hunt in her 1993 research. Although some of these suggestions may seem most appropriate for children, many are useful "mood changers" for people of all ages. A clown, for instance, seems to bring smiles quickly to children and adults alike. Playfulness is not for children only but rather a helpful means of maintaining well-being for people of all ages. Get to know what appeals to the person in your care. Take a risk and try some humorous "mood changers"; chances are great that you *both* will have some fun.

Creativity and Self-Expression

A person needs to express individual feelings and responses to life in order to feel whole and healthy. Expressing "the self" is important to being oneself. Gerontologist and sociologist Nancy J. Osgood explained in 1993 that creative activities—art, creative writing, music, poetry, drama, and dance—offer opportunity for creative expression, personal exploration and growth, and release of tension. Emphasizing the importance of creative leisure experiences, she went on to say that creative activities are fun. They provide a necessary balance to the strains and tensions and mundane tasks of day-to-day living. We temporarily forget our troubles and cares and relax. Creative involvement can almost magically restore, refresh, revitalize, and re-create an individual. We all have a need for freedom, joy, pleasure, beauty, aesthetics, and passion—these the arts can fulfill.

Such refreshment and revitalization are important in the caregiving process. Being creative through the arts is an important means of self-expression for both the caregiver and the person receiving care—independently and jointly. Try to find the avenues for self-expression that suit your particular interests. The "self-expressive activities and hobbies" section of the Checklist of Leisure Favorites can be helpful in determining useful and enjoyable activities in this area. There are many possibilities for being creative, both in the arts and beyond.

Edna

Edna always claimed she was not creative. Yet, when her volunteer visitor, Savanna, completed her Checklist of Leisure Favorites, she discovered that eighty-four-year-old Edna had many interests that helped her be creative: she baked marvelous rolls and breads, cooked most foods "from scratch," embroidered pillowcases, crocheted beautiful doilies, and had a lovely singing voice. When Savanna pointed out these creative activities to her, Edna replied, "Yes, but I can't draw a straight line."

Edna is not alone in how she views creativity. Many others, like her, may have creative daily activities but don't think of themselves as creative. Creativity and self-expression take many forms and include far more than drawing or the other arts. Fixing things, baking bread, making pickles, dancing, are all outlets for self-expression. Some people use traditional activities while others use nontraditional activities (discussed in Chapter 1) and daily living as a means to be creative. Self-expression results from such common enjoyments as: singing old songs, doodling, making a terrific salad, growing plants, caring for a pet, arranging flowers, carving wood, taking photos. Whenever people are being unique, making something their own way or doing things with their own bent, they are expressing themselves creatively.

Dana

In the midst of living with AIDS, Dana spent many days at home. Her sister Renee was her primary caregiver, although home health aides assisted several hours each week. Dana required hours of rest each day, but when she was awake she found solace in a variety of self-expressive activities that helped her manage pain, stress, and frustration. At least once each day she wrote in her journal, even if an entry just said she didn't feel like writing that day. She used her journal to hold not only precious words, but poems, doodles, and colorful drawings. She discovered time went by quickly and with less pain when she engrossed herself in her creative works. Sometimes she was quiet and other times she played music to help express what was on her mind and in her heart. When she envisioned images along with the music, she liked to make drawings of her visualizations in her journal. She and Renee had many conversations about the drawings and sometimes they wrote poems together; sometimes they sang together. The words and pictures and songs helped them connect with each other's spirits, tackle their feelings and worries, and talk about fears as well as blessings. Dana's journal became quite an elaborate account of their lives and what she was feeling. She found comfort in her self-expression.

We can see that Dana used a variety of activities to express her emotions for various purposes, such as distraction and stress management. Artist and author Beverly Baer believes strongly in the healing qualities of creative expression and pointed out in 1985 that the expressive arts make it possible to express deep thoughts and feelings in socially acceptable outlets. She further explained that feelings of stress, fear, guilt, anger, and despair are often suppressed and difficult to put into words. Sometimes nonverbal expressions through art, music, song, dance, or drama serve to express those feelings more adequately. Also, it may be especially difficult for a person who is dependent on a caregiver to release negative feelings without jeopardizing the caregiving relationship; creative expression gives an acceptable outlet for such feelings without endangering communication.

Creative expression is often a solitary activity. As a caregiver your main responsibility in this area may be obtaining supplies and materials to support expressive activities and to encourage self-expression. These are important roles. In the case of Dana, though, we see not only that her creative expressions helped her with her own feelings, but that sharing her creative products with her sister led them to a deeper level of communication. Writing in 1991 about the healing qualities of imagery and creativity, Kathy Goff and Paul E. Torrance of the Georgia Studies of Creative Behavior emphasized that creative activities give people opportunities to communicate with each other as well as with themselves. Similar opportunities may arise with your care recipient if he or she is willing to share aspects of the experience with you.

Creative experiences also help to reduce stress and improve ability to cope with difficult circumstances. The "timeless" experience that comes with paying full attention to creative activity is useful in diverting attention from pain and difficulties. After the outpouring of expression, many people feel a release and sense of deep calm. In the case of Dana, she found comfort in her creative endeavors. Your care receiver may also find this kind of activity uplifting and relaxing.

Whether simple or elaborate, keeping a journal can be a useful means of expressing feelings. Dana's journal held a variety of words, poems, doodles, and drawings. A journal can become whatever the owner wants it to be. It may be a notebook for writing daily or occasional entries, or it may be a large file of combined mediums of self-expression. Many people find keeping a journal a satisfying activity and a way to keep track of and "make sense" of, or understand, life experiences.

Music, too, is an enjoyable and helpful means of self-expression. Listening to music can be both comforting and stimulating. Many people listen to their favorite music to help them manage stress. Singing adds another dimension to the music experience. In 1984 music therapist Lucanne Magill Bailey explained that when we select songs such as "You've Got a Friend," "Take Me Home, Country Roads," "How Great Thou Art," or "Let It Be Me" we can express specific feelings. Bailey also stressed that singing not only sets the stage for pleasure and release of tension but offers opportunity to reminisce, express feelings, and think about issues like loss, life, death, and peace. Through songs we can communicate happiness, loneliness, problems, and hopes; we can also build relationships. If you and the other person like to sing, try singing together. It just may turn out to be a positive leisure experience for you both. (As noted in the article "Singing with Mom" in Chapter 1 of this book.) You can even sing while you do other things. Some people find that if they sing while they work, their tasks become easier and get done in less time.

Not only can self-expressive activities be helpful to the care recipient, but you as caregiver can benefit from your *own* creative expressions. You, too, can find comfort, a sense of calm, and stress reduction through leisure moments engaged in creative endeavors. When feelings are pent up inside, use a paper and pen to say on paper what you are feeling, or make a giant doodle that says it all, or draw the feelings in color to show just how you feel inside. You don't need to save the products if you don't want to. Just getting the feelings out and putting them on paper may be enough. On the other hand, you might feel like keeping a file of your doodles or writings or even feel like framing a drawing as a reminder of a special point in time. Let yourself as well as your care receiver experience the benefits of self-expressive activities.

Hobbies

A hobby is something a person likes to do in spare time. It may be very simple or quite complex, but usually a hobby involves ongoing activity and enduring interest. Examples include photography, needle crafts, gardening and caring for plants, computer games, running, drawing, collecting things, playing a musical instrument, writing letters, reading, studying topics of interest, and dismantling or assembling things. A hobby goes on without ever coming to a complete end, although specific phases may come to completion. The ongoing nature of a hobby makes it especially useful as something to look forward to and keep going back to. When we engage in a hobby, time flies because we are engrossed in enjoyable activity, and we often experience a "timeless," pleasurable feeling. Large chunks of time may go by without our ever looking at the clock or thinking about our responsibilities. Hobbies can divert attention from pain and concerns. For these many reasons, hobbies are especially useful to a person during times of illness and disability.

Jacob

Jacob made lawn furniture and birdhouses for years. Now that he needed supervision due to frailty and poor eyesight, he no longer was able to manage the woodworking equipment. Adam, a volunteer visitor, enjoyed woodworking also, and he came by to visit Jacob two or three times each month. Jacob didn't speak very much, so visiting was difficult, but Adam decided that didn't matter, and maybe the visits would go better if they did some activity together. So, when Adam visited, he brought along pieces of wood to be sanded. Jacob still had it in him! He could sand wood quite well, even though his eyesight was limited. He seemed to enjoy the feel of the wood. Jacob was able to do some of the initial sanding, and Adam added the finishing touches. The sanding project was a good way to keep Jacob involved in at least part of his old hobby. It gave them something to do during visits, and they both felt a sense of accomplishment.

Since Jacob had worked with wood much of his life, he was familiar with the feel of wood, and how to sand it. He no longer was able to complete all the tasks involved, but he could still contribute his part to woodworking projects. Just as Adam figured out a part of the whole that Jacob still could do, you can think about the skills of your care receiver and try to find small ways for him or her to be self-expressive or contribute to a larger project.

A former cook who has lost strength to walk around the kitchen to make a meal may still be able to sit at the table and mix ingredients in a bowl or cut fruit or wash the vegetables, or add mushrooms and onions to a pizza. A gardener may no longer be able to work outside in a garden but can enjoy potted plants on the porch, deck, or patio or care for indoor plants which require daily attention and nurturing. A photography buff may no longer get out and about to take photos but may be able to sort, label, and display photos from the past or take pictures of indoor activity in the home. A golfer unable to walk an entire golf course may still be able to ride in a golf cart and play three holes, or take a few shots on the putting green, or hit some balls in the backyard. I have a friend who has made arrangements with the manager of a golf course to ride the pathways of the course in a golf cart, at low-traffic hours and observing golfers' courtesy, just to enjoy the open space and beauty of the golf course. The idea is to make the most of former activities, even if it means using only a few remaining skills for short moments of meaningful activity.

As a caregiver, consider how you can make modifications in your *own* hobbies and leisure pursuits to suit your current lifestyle situation. In your caregiving role it may be difficult to pursue your hobbies, continue a former exercise program, or keep in contact with your friends. The same principle of modification and adaptation applies to you. Give serious thought to how you can maintain even "little bits" of your former enjoyable activities to find pleasurable moments now to maintain good health and life balance when you need it desperately.

Perhaps you can give yourself a few minutes each day for a telephone visit with a friend or schedule a minimum of ten minutes for a walk. If you cannot leave the house because of your care receiver's condition, you might exercise with a videotape or do your own movements to music. If you find it impossible to do needle crafts that you enjoyed before you became a caregiver, perhaps you can at least look through related magazines or catalogs and plan ahead for projects you have in mind for the future. It is important that you maintain at least some of your past interests in order to keep a sense of your own identity—your own unique self. If you have a connection to other caregivers, you help them, and they can help you, come up with ideas of how to keep yourselves "leisurely alive" in spite of your caregiving roles.

Dwight

Dwight's family farm had a wooded area with walnut trees. Every fall, family members gathered sacks full of walnuts to be cracked during the winter and used among family, friends, and neighbors in favorite baked goods. Dwight's hobby, for years, was being in charge of the operation and cracking the walnuts. His habit was to sit in the evenings with a pan full of walnuts and crack them while he listened to the radio or watched TV.

After being diagnosed with cancer, Dwight continued his walnut cracking as though nothing had changed. It gave him daily purpose and a connection to his precancer life. Family and friends depended on him to provide their supply of walnuts as usual, so he wasn't about to let them down. When time came to gather nuts in the fall, this time he let the rest of the family do the job without him; but, with or without pain, Dwight cracked at least a few nuts every day until the day he died. His hobby served him well, and through it he continued to be of service.

Often a hobby provides reason to wake up every day and do something that feels worthwhile, which was the case for Dwight. Most people want to feel useful, even when care from others is necessary. You can build self-esteem by encouraging meaningful ways for the person in your care to be of service and feel useful. Professor of leisure studies Arnold H. Grossman of New York University noted in 1996 that, for some people and in some cultures, playful activity is considered frivolous and contrary to work and cultural ethics, whereas being of service or volunteering is considered meaningful activity. Perhaps your care receiver is a person who did not cultivate leisure activities yet had meaningful activity in other ways—perhaps through volunteer service to others, or feeling productive by making or fixing things. Consider how you can help him or her still feel useful. Promoting a hobby is a good way to start.

If a person does not have a hobby, there are new things to learn even at a time of illness or disability. A thirteen-year-old boy, hospitalized with cancer, learned to draw cartoons by watching the therapeutic recreation specialist make cartoon posters. She offered to teach him, and he eagerly took "lessons." In a few days he had a new skill and a hobby that occupied his time in the hospital bed. In fact, being an enterprising teenager, he saw the chance to make some money for treats—even in the hospital. Daily he worked on drawings that he compiled into creative little booklets for sale among hospital personnel. He made enough money to support his sweet tooth and kept drawing until the day he died. Hospital staff still have his booklets and cherish their memories of him. His hobby provided him with a reason to wake up every day and do something for others, too.

It may take some time to get to know someone, even a family member, well enough to creatively figure out how to use interests and talents to be of service. Be patient. As you get to know someone, and as you continue to gather information, you will find ways to build meaningful activity into everyday enjoyment and discover how to help the person feel a part of things through service activity.

One of my friends takes her self-assigned job seriously as she daily cuts coupons from newspapers and magazines to leave in a basket at the door of her neighborhood grocery store so her neighbors can save money. Another friend calls three other homebound people in the community every day to check on their health and share a visit. These are useful leisure-time hobbies and may be "jobs" suited to the person in your care.

Being of Service to Others

Alice

Alice, an older person with brittle diabetes, lived in a foster care home so she would have full-time supervision. She was quite artistic throughout her life. Recently, she began making her own greeting cards by cutting out pictures and verses from used cards that she had saved and pasting them onto paper that she folded to fit into envelopes. People of all ages found her cards attractive. Alice entered a few of her cards in the "Recycled Item" category at the county fair and won grand prize. Word spread about her prize and skill. A local boy scout troop made an appointment to have their troop meet with her in hopes she would teach them to recycle greeting cards. She was amazed beyond belief. Her simple hobby not only won her recognition (and money, too), but young boys wanted to learn something from her. She graciously accommodated them and charmed them in the process. Now, they continue to visit her from time to time to show off *their* cards.

Alice had more to teach others than she realized. She was surprised that anyone would want to learn about her recycled greeting cards. She enjoyed making them herself but never considered that she could help others by teaching them her skill. It is very possible that your care recipient, too, has more to share than he or she thinks. You might arrange simple teaching and learning situations if the person wants to be of service this way. A good starting point is to learn things from each other. It is likely each of you has a skill you can teach the other and have some fun doing it. An interesting way to fold napkins, how to crochet bedroom slippers, how to blow on long grass to produce a whistling sound, how to skip stones across water, how to properly use cutting shears, how to make a family-favorite food, how to recognize edible mushrooms . . . the list is endless. Remember, the fun here is to share with each other some of the many skills each of you has. And, if you say you can't do anything, think again. Everyone has at least a few skills to share. Think about it and take a chance on having some fun sharing with each other. As caregiver, you might break the ice and be the "teacher" first; then, ask the other person to teach you something, and take turns, perhaps sharing something each week. If the skill you want to teach requires special supplies or equipment that are not available, then try describing for the other person how it is done or draw a diagram to explain.

Look for other possible "students" to learn your care receiver's skill. Other family members, neighbors, volunteers, children at a nearby school, or a scout troop may be candidates to learn something the person has to offer. Sometimes there are specialties within family traditions that are, sadly, lost with the passing of the family members who have those special skills. It may be meaningful for everyone involved if those skills and specialties are passed on. The sense of service is keen for the person passing along the information, and the skills gained allow family traditions to continue.

It may not be possible to carry out the actual teaching and learning experience as described above. You also can help the person write down directions, recipes, stories, and advice to pass on to others. Make an audiotape or videotape to help pass along key information about how to do or make things which others might want to learn. If someone is too timid for cameras and tape recorders, see if they will allow you to write down their special strategies so that others can learn. Everyone has significant, unique ways of expressing the "self" and distinctive contributions to pass on to others.

A friend of mine whose mother died from cancer tells the story of her family realizing that no one but her mother knew how to make lefsa (Swedish potato bread). The week before she died, after her two sons and daughter begged her to teach them her specialty, she got up from her bed, came to the kitchen in her robe and bandaged arm, and supervised her grown children in learning to carry on their family tradition, all the while enjoying wonderful laughter and freedom from pain. What a fabulous way to be of service to her family and feel important. Besides, when my friend tells the story, the smile on her face tells the story of how important that memory is to her and her family. They made the moments count!

Summary

Each person is unique, and leisure experiences are useful in expressing individuality. Humor and playful activities are enjoyable ways to stabilize moods and lighten daily living. Even in the caregiving process, the creative arts and a variety of other traditional and nontraditional expressive activities support emotional health, enjoyment, and peace of mind. Hobbies and service-oriented projects provide opportunities to engage in meaningful activity and be helpful to others.

Emotional and Expressive Activity Ideas

acting	arts and crafts
baking	being silly
bragging	building things
clowning	collecting things
cooking	creating a business
dancing	decorating cakes, cookies
decorating for holidays	drawing
dressing up	growing something
making a costume	making a wish list
making decorations	making greeting cards
making love	painting
photography	planning a party
playing music	rearranging furniture
sewing	singing
sorting stuff	teaching something to someone
telling jokes	telling stories
writing letters	writing poetry
writing stories	woodworking
other _____	_____

CHAPTER SIX

Social Activity

BENEFITS
Social activities can put one in contact with people, plants, pets, the community, and provide occasions to meet people, talk, share interests, make and nurture relationships, join in activities, and build group cohesiveness.

We are social beings with complex needs to associate with other people and with our world. Leisure activities involve a host of social elements that can help us make and maintain relationships. In this chapter you will find information about the following:

☆ Integrating contacts with people, plants, and pets into the caregiving process
☆ Maintaining associations with clubs and organizations
☆ Planning "special" events
☆ Celebrating holidays
☆ Planning and implementing enjoyable outings

Making Connections

Many leisure activities lend themselves to making meaningful connections. Often the caregiving process makes it difficult for both the caregiver and care receiver to stay connected to family, friends, neighbors, and community. Social activities and special events can help to prevent isolation and provide healthful outcomes. In 1994 gerontologist Rachelle A. Dorfman brought together evidence showing that social relationships can positively influence health. For example, social relationships have been shown to help people more quickly recover from illness by enhancing their immunity. In the caregiving process, a person's social network may get smaller because of the person's illness, disability, or confinement. With planning and creativity, though, the caregiver can blend enjoyable (and healing) social contacts into leisure moments.

Including Other People

Sometimes, when we become caregivers or volunteer visitors, we think we can meet all the social needs of the other person. And yet, he or she almost certainly needs *other* people, as well, especially family, friends, and neighbors. Activities that include other people can be fun for everyone involved. The caregiver will find the "family and friends" portion of the Checklist of Leisure Favorites useful in identifying people who are important to the person receiving care. Another way to find out is to reminisce with the person receiving care, or talk with the person's family and friends, and ask whose company he or she has enjoyed recently and through the years.

Because there are unique factors in your care receiver's situation, you will want to think carefully through the details of visiting others or bringing others into the caregiving environment. Different people will react differently to the person's situation. Some visitors will do better if you give them some information before the visit: about the person's health, appearance, or whatever seems appropriate. Ask visitors to let you know when they will be stopping by so you can also prepare your care receiver for the visit. It is best to prepare everyone involved for visits rather than expect anyone to adjust quickly to surprises. Also, when a visit *isn't* convenient, be sure to say so.

Lydia

Lydia was back home after recuperating from a stroke. Her husband, Ed, found himself in the new role of household manager. With Lydia's help and consultation from their children, he adjusted well. However, he realized they needed more visitors to keep up with Lydia's social needs. So, Ed contacted the Social Concerns Committee at their church and asked for a volunteer visitor for Lydia. When Sue was contacted, she immediately knew that this was something she wanted to do.

When Sue volunteered to visit one afternoon each week, she expected to satisfy Lydia's social need for visitors. But during every visit, Lydia complained about being lonely and never seeing her friends and neighbors. They rarely stopped by anymore since her stroke. It seemed many of Lydia's friends and neighbors were afraid to face her now. They were unsure about what had happened to her. They were afraid they might say or do the wrong thing. They were uncomfortable being with her.

Sue decided to try to arrange some visits with Lydia and a few of her friends. She called the friends and explained Lydia's current condition, how they could best communicate with her, and how much she still needed them. Sue accepted the fact that some people just couldn't feel comfortable with Lydia now, and rather than making them feel guilty, she focused on the friends who still did want to spend time with Lydia.

Sue helped potential visitors understand that Lydia did want to see them and could understand them well, but that she could not say long sentences or follow complicated questions. Sue gave the friends these suggestions about visiting: because Lydia found it easiest to talk about things she could see and touch, they might focus attention on items around the house; or they might talk about their interests—such as gardening and cooking—or reminisce about good times; and Sue told them it would be important to keep visits short because Lydia tired easily.

When friends visited, Lydia liked to show them the most recent photos of her family members. One of her friends usually brought pictures, too, so she could update Lydia on her family as well. One of Lydia's best visits took place when a neighbor stopped by with an armful of dahlias she cut from her flower garden. She brought a vase, and she and Lydia spent a half hour cutting and arranging the flowers to Lydia's liking. The arrangement may not have won an award at the garden club, but being involved in an activity with her friend was enjoyable for them both.

Lydia always liked to offer a cup of coffee to her guests, just as she had over the years, and she enjoyed supervising Sue while Sue set up the tray of cream and sugar, cups, saucers, and napkins—selected by Lydia. Sue also found that Lydia was more comfortable with visitors when her hair was combed and she was wearing earrings (since she was used to wearing them both at home and away) and she made sure that visitors didn't find Lydia in her robe or night clothes. She knew how important good grooming had been in Lydia's life, and now she was careful to help her look her best in spite of her current limitations. This made Lydia feel better and made her visitors more at ease.

Sue tried to accommodate the needs of Lydia and her visitors by looking ahead and trying to anticipate what would work best. One thing she noticed was that *short* visits usually worked best for everyone. And, depending upon your care recipient's health or condition, short visits may be all that's possible or advisable. They can give others the opportunity to visit and maintain the relationship yet prevent uncomfortable strain. Watch for signs of fatigue and be prepared to suggest politely that this visit had better end, with the possibility for another visit later in the week or month. And, if your care receiver is only up to a short visit, be sure to let the visitor know in advance.

Just as Sue did with Lydia, you can plan simple activities to keep visits interesting. Arrange for care receiver and visitors to do such things together as arranging flowers, looking at photos, putting together puzzles, or sharing a cup of tea. This does not mean that you need to keep everyone busy all the time. But it's interesting to see how often a visit is made more comfortable when people have something to do while visiting. For example, when my family plays cards, we sit down for a hand or two of cards, and then while someone is dealing the cards, a topic of conversation comes up. Thereafter the game is delayed until that topic runs out and we resume a round or two of cards followed by more talk, then some cards, more talk, and so on. Observers might be hard pressed to determine whether this is card playing or family visiting. Indeed, it is both. We talk much more freely with cards in our hands—with something to do—than we do sitting "eyeball to eyeball" in intensive personal interchange. That is true for many people, not just our family.

Draw the attention of visitors and the care receiver to things they can see and relate to. If conversation lags and people seem to feel uncomfortable, they will find topics of common interest based on real things in their midst. You can steer their attention to such things as household items, greeting cards, jewelry, catalogs, house plants, pictures in magazines, newspaper articles, photos of family or friends. You need not come up with exotic activities or novel conversation. Simple activities are often the best.

You can look forward to a visit by involving the person in simple preparations, such as putting crackers on a plate, folding napkins, buttering bread for sandwiches, or just supervising the preparations. By sharing in the preparations (if possible) the care receiver can look forward to the visit. Sometimes the anticipation of an event is just as satisfying as the actual event; sometimes more so.

Keep account of which visitors and which activities are most successful; that way you can repeat the successes. By observing the care recipient's level of comfort during a visit and noting the conversations, smiles, and laughter, you will be able to determine how much he or she enjoyed the people and the experience. Be ready to invite back the people whose visits were most enjoyed.

Keeping in Touch with Other Living Things

We can have relationships with plants and pets as well as with other people. In fact, during a time of illness or disability, it may be easier for someone to relate to a plant or a pet than to deal with human visitors. Plants and pets don't ask threatening questions; nor do they have any expectations. Animals respond to love with their own loving ways of licking, barking or purring, playing, or resting on a companion's lap. Pets provide much-needed affection and affirming touch during times of illness or disability. Petting a dog or a cat is a good way to feel warmth and affection. It is important that a person receiving care have real opportunities to touch, hug, kiss, and give and receive affection— whether with family and friends or with animals.

Rosa

Rosa's daughter Donna was her full-time caregiver now that Rosa's cancer had progressed, and Rosa required ongoing supervision. Rosa and Donna lived in Donna's apartment, although Rosa grew up on a farm and had raised her family in a large house in town. Rosa had a number of pet dogs when she grew up and when she raised her own family. Rocky, an aging cocker spaniel, was her current pet and heart-warming companion.

Donna decided Rocky would be an important member of her caregiving team. She noticed the dog's presence seemed to cheer Rosa and keep her connected to reality. The dog was able to put a smile on Rosa's face any time of the day or night; he snuggled on the sofa with Rosa and let her pet him quietly. They seemed to comfort each other.

Donna thought about her mother's life and remembered how she enjoyed gardening and raising plants. This wasn't a good time to raise a garden outdoors or get involved in farming; their apartment was too modest for that; time and health were barriers, too. However, Donna had heard that every kitchen cupboard has a variety of things that grow from seed. One afternoon she went to the cupboard and came up with a few things that might sprout. There were whole cloves, fennel seeds, celery seeds, caraway seeds, and popcorn.

One afternoon when Rosa felt up to it, she and Donna sat at the kitchen table and enjoyed some planting. In paper cups, they put a few inches of potting soil, then a few of each kind of seed, labeled the cups according to the seeds, watered the soil, and set the cups on the windowsill for light and heat. Although Rosa could not pay attention very long, she was able to stick with the planting project and seemed to enjoy it. Planting a few simple seeds in paper cups was quite different from raising a whole garden but still gave Rosa the opportunity to plant and nurture something. In the days that followed, Donna and Rosa looked at the paper cup planters every morning and watered them as needed. Then, Lo and Behold! Day by day sprouts came through and they could watch the little plants grow.

Pets and plants can provide unconditional love. They don't care if a person's hair is combed or if the house is clean. They just want to give and receive love and attention. The unconditional love of a pet may be just the spark a person needs when feeling blue or when others have too high expectations. Petting an animal brings comfort and companionship: a real relationship at a time when other relationships may be difficult to maintain. Pets and plants help pass time pleasurably and provide distraction from troubles, pain, or boredom.

Pets also provide a variety of other positive outcomes for their companions. In their 1989 study of the effect of pets on the health of older persons, Dan Lago and associates in the College of Health and Human

Development at Pennsylvania State University found that pets help to improve morale and therefore have positive impact on health—an outcome supported by the *Mayo Clinic Health Letter* in 1995. In one study, pet owners reported fewer doctor contacts over one year than persons without pets, and the pets seemed to help their owners in times of stress. Animals seem to bring optimism to people and quickly produce smiles. Activities specialist James R. Dowling noted in 1995 that, since cats and dogs are familiar to many people, they easily spark stories for reminiscing, as well.

A live-in pet does not always suit the caregiving situation, however. But pet owners may be willing to bring a pet to visit. Friends, neighbors, or family members may have pets they can bring to the home. Also, volunteer visitors may be available to bring pets to visit someone who is homebound. In some communities, you can call on organizations such as Therapy Dogs International, Inc. (see the Related Resources section of this book) made up of local pet owners who have trained their animals to serve persons with illness or disability.

Although plants may not move about and play like pets, they, too, are living things, and gardening can be simple and fun—outdoors or indoors. Gardening is one of the most popular leisure-time activities, and in the words of program development consultant Pamela L. McKee, gardening is "an equal opportunity joy" that provides a certain "spiritual medicine" in the wonder of watching flowers and vegetables grow and produce marvelous color, fragrances, and flavors.

For those who are unable to be outside in the garden, plants can be grown indoors in cups, pots, and window boxes. Seeds, cuttings, and small plants can be obtained from flower and garden shops, nurseries, and seed catalogs. It is even possible to enjoy the plants that grow from common "kitchen seeds" such as popcorn, whole cloves, fennel seeds, celery seeds, caraway seeds, dried beans and peas. But be sure you don't try to plant seeds that are cracked, chopped, ground, or split. Only whole seeds will sprout, and since they have been dormant a long time, they may have a low rate of germination. You will be even more successful planting actual vegetable, herb, or flower seeds which can be obtained from stores and nurseries especially during early weeks of the growing season. If you plant herbs, you can enjoy the additional features of their pleasant aromas and then add their zesty flavors to your foods.

Also, orange seeds, apple seeds, and grapefruit seeds will sprout and grow if you allow them several days to dry before planting them. Give it a try. You will be amazed. Some years ago I dried, for about two weeks, a few seeds from a grapefruit I ate for breakfast. Then I planted the seeds in a paper cup in which I had punched small holes at the bottom for drainage and put the cup in a saucer on the windowsill for adequate sunlight. After many days of keeping the seeds moist, two of them sprouted. When they were growing nicely and had a few leaves, I transplanted them to a small flower pot where they flourished. The deep green leaves were lovely among my other house plants. Of course, raising them in my apartment didn't give them the conditions they needed to ever bear grapefruit, but I enjoyed their beauty for a long time.

If you do not have paper cups and soil available, you can sprout seeds in paper towels that you keep wet and warm over a period of a few days. Sometimes it is fun just to watch seeds germinate and sprout and be amazed at the process. You can sprout alfalfa seeds this way and then eat the sprouts in salads. In addition, bulbs, such as tulip and crocus bulbs, can be "forced" into blooming indoors in pots even during winter months. Plant them in a pot of potting soil and water them to keep the soil moist. Keep them warm and they will sprout and soon bloom, giving you wonderful color.

In the spring of the year, many stores carry bedding plants of both flowers and vegetables. It is a good time to get out (if possible) to see the assorted plants and enjoy their colors and fragrances. Then, selecting just a few plants to take home to plant in a special pot, window box, patio planter, or outdoor garden can be especially satisfying and give both you and the person in your care something to watch and talk about for a long time. If the outing is impossible for your care recipient, you can make the selection and bring home a few appropriate plants to enjoy together.

For you as caregiver, too, living things such as plants and pets can provide color and beauty as well as opportunity to relate to something besides human needs. Treat yourself to flowers from time to time. Don't wait for someone to give them to you or think the care receiver is the only one who should be getting flowers at this time. You deserve to care for *yourself* as well as others. A few flowers, a charming plant, or a few goldfish won't cost a fortune but can brighten your days.

Luke

Luke, a twenty-seven-year-old man with moderate developmental disability, lived in an apartment and worked at a sheltered workshop during morning hours. Carlos, a student volunteer caregiver from a local college, visited Luke on weekends to take him out for leisure-time activities and help him with his cooking and hygiene skills. Carlos used the Checklist of Leisure Favorites to find out some of Luke's interests and discovered that he loved pets. So, Carlos brought his dog, Pepper, along for a visit. Luke and Pepper were immediate friends.

Luke let Carlos know that he, too, wanted to have a dog. Luke's two-room apartment didn't lend itself to such a pet, but because Luke clearly loved animals Carlos decided to ask Luke's case worker about the matter. The answer was that some small pet, such as a gerbil or fish, might work, but a large animal needing extensive care was out of the question for Luke. His nurturing skills were not adequate to support a large animal. Carlos decided to bring Luke to his apartment to see his fish tank. He had four goldfish that required little care, yet gave him much pleasure. He showed Luke how he feeds and cares for his fish. Luke showed much interest. He also admired two small plants Carlos had in his window.

Carlos decided to take Luke on an outing to a pet shop, where they looked at dogs, of course, and a variety of other pets. The shop owner described what each animal would need and how to care for it. Carlos focused Luke's attention on fish and fish tanks. By the time they left, Luke had enjoyed visiting several pets and decided he wanted a fish tank like the one Carlos had in his apartment. Carlos promised to help Luke prepare space in the apartment for the tank and help him set it up.

A week later they picked up the tank and several fish at the pet store and proceeded to set up the system in Luke's apartment. Carlos brought Luke a plant to celebrate the occasion. They set that on the window ledge above the tank. Luke was very excited. Over the next months, Luke spent hours watching his fish, feeding them, and looking after their welfare. Carlos kept up his visits, with Pepper present too, and together they cleaned, maintained, and enjoyed Luke's new pets.

Sometimes, a visit to pet or plant stores may be sufficient to provide meaningful contact with living things. A stroll through a greenhouse or flower shop may satisfy a plant lover's need to be in touch with plants and flowers. Visiting the animal exhibits at a county fair, going to a pet shop or to a pet show, or visiting an animal farm can also serve this need.

Pets and plants provide opportunity to nurture and care about something besides oneself. Just because a person is ill or disabled doesn't mean he or she has lost the need to be needed. There are very few opportunities for a person receiving care to do something for someone else. A plant or a pet can be a good reason to get up every morning. If the plants must be watered and the drapes pulled for light or the fish must be fed or the dog needs to be walked, or the bird feeder outside the window is empty and must be filled to attract birds for daily enjoyment—these are good reasons to be in a specific place at a definite time doing something important.

If your caregiving situation does not allow for pets and plants in the environment, TV programs or videotapes about nature and plants and animals may satisfy this interest. For some people an aquarium with a variety of fish or a simple fish bowl with a goldfish or two can be the source of much entertainment and relaxation, but watching a fish videotape is another alternative. Therapeutic recreation specialists Mary M. DeSchriver and Carol C. Riddick in 1990 conducted an interesting study in which they found that watching an aquarium or a fish video can lower pulse rates and stress. In fact, watching a videotape of an aquarium may have a greater positive impact on stress than watching a live aquarium. Videotapes of fish or other animals, then, offer another means to stay in touch with living things. (Although viewing a fish videotape may serve a need to reduce stress, it will not serve other needs discussed above, such as nurturing and caring for something besides oneself.)

As the caregiver, you could take on all the responsibility not only for your care receiver but also for all the plants, pets, and children in the household. Instead of automatically assuming all those duties, however, you might consider which ones can be carried out successfully by the other person, and then share the responsibility. If the person receiving care is confined to bed, you might set plants by the bedside to be watered there; or keep the goldfish bowl handy so he or she can sprinkle fish food on the water and watch the daily feeding. These tasks may seem very small, but for the care receiver they are moments to look forward to, and they allow him or her to enjoy making a small contribution to another life.

Not everyone loves plants and animals, though. Some people are afraid of animals because of past negative experiences or because the animals' quick movements and unpredictable nature make them nervous. Others may be allergic to animals or plants. Be sensitive to such needs and individual differences. Don't "force" experiences with plants or pets—or any other experiences for that matter. Rather, try to identify genuine interest and be vigilant about safety in this area.

Maintaining Contact with Clubs and Organizations

Some persons receiving care have enjoyed years of interesting interactions with the community through membership in clubs and organizations. Unfortunately, when illness or disability prevent ongoing participation, the organization often sends a get-well card and the connection is broken, not because no one cares but because few know what to do to maintain meaningful contact. Sometimes poor health, pain, fatigue, or embarrassment leave the care recipient content to end the contact. If the person does have interest in maintaining connections with clubs and organizations, though, doing so can bring much joy to the homebound member.

A member willing to serve as a "buddy" can be the communicating link between the person at home and the organization. Duties include being the friendly representative of the group, stopping by after a meeting to give information about transactions and club activities, and relating to the group the ideas and opinions of the homebound member. The role of "buddy" can be passed from one member to another, giving everyone an opportunity to visit.

The "buddy" also can bring to the care receiver small tasks to be accomplished at home (if health and interest permit), such as stuffing envelopes and addressing them for a club mailing, counting money, ordering items needed by members, conducting a telephone survey, cutting out decorations for special events, working on a newsletter, or finding information on the Internet. Given the ability, interest, and willingness on the part of the member at home and thoughtful effort among organization members, it is possible to maintain ties with community groups.

Special Occasions

A celebration is a special time when ordinary chores are set aside to acknowledge something special that took place in the past or something special we anticipate in the future. A graduation party signifies the reaching of a milestone; it is a time set aside to recognize a person's academic efforts and look forward to another stage of life. A wedding reception celebrates the beginning of a couple's life together; a national holiday is set aside to recognize the historical contribution made by a person or event. In his 1969 book *The Feast of Fools*, eminent philosopher Harvey Cox noted that human beings are the only animals that celebrate because only human beings have the ability to ponder the significance of a celebration. Other animals play, but celebrating is an especially "human" thing to do. Special occasions of all sorts give us reason to celebrate, whether it is a birthday, an anniversary, a graduation, or a national or religious holiday.

Celebrations are important in the normal course of living, but when life changes bring the need for caregiving, it is easy to feel as though nothing is "normal" anymore. At such times we may feel a sense of loss over the way things used to be, especially when special events such as holidays roll around. Yet, it is possible to celebrate and make special events, holidays, and outings meaningful in spite of life changes. You can take a party to the person with dinner and drinks in the bedroom, as suggested by Andrea Sankar in her book *Dying at Home*, or bring a cap and gown home for an in-home graduation ceremony complete with graduate, family, and friends joining in a graduation march through the house and a "commencement speech" given by a friend or family member. It will take some creativity to come up with new or different ways to celebrate, but it can be done.

A family I know couldn't manage their usual Fourth of July weekend at the lake due to caregiving responsibilities, so instead they invited family members to their own home, called the backyard the lake, told guests to look after their own needs and not expect to be waited on, grilled every meal and ate picnic style outdoors, put on swim suits and ran through the sprinkler, and played outdoor games. The kids even set a washtub with water in the backyard and took their fishing poles to the deck of the house where they had casting contests to see who could cast into the "lake" below. The best part was that the care receiver was part of the celebration, and they all had a Fourth of July they'll always remember. With a little creativity, any event can become "special."

If the person in your care can participate only partially in the meaning of an event due to physical or mental impairment, it is still wise to make the moment special in some way, just as you would with anyone else. Create the air of celebration in your usual way. It is the "human" thing to do for the other participants and for the care receiver. The variety of foods, refreshments, decorations, colors, or company will provide sensory stimulation, a positive environment, and generate good feelings, all of which are healthy circumstances for any human being.

If the person in your care has dementia, you will want to protect him or her from extensive activity that could cause sensory overload (discussed earlier in Chapter 4) and fatigue. It is best to avoid placing the person in the midst of a great deal of noise and many people. The idea is to give the person a pleasant experience, so having the person with dementia share in only a portion of the celebration may be more enjoyable than being present for it all.

Making the event special will give *you* a change of pace, too. You can make even the planning and preparations into leisure activities. If you plan ahead you might call friends or family to visit for the occasion, make simple decorations, fold napkins in a certain way, and prepare foods to fit the event. You can make a "group project" out of preparations by involving guests in some of the tasks, too. Each of these activities is a potential nontraditional leisure activity in itself (discussed in Chapter 1). If the preparations seem to add to your burden, however, they will not be leisurely. So, include only what is comfortable and feels like fun. More is not always better! "Special" does not necessarily mean "elaborate" when it comes to having a special event. "Simple" can be just as enjoyable as "elaborate," sometimes more so. The final celebration is just one step of the whole event. Be sure to try to enjoy *all* the steps in the process.

In many groups and families there are topics of conversation that frequently end in everyone agreeing, "Yes, that would be special. We should do that sometime." And then, time goes by and no one schedules that "special" something, and it never becomes a reality; it remains just a wish. If you hear yourself, family, or friends saying, "Oh, let's do that sometime," go to the calendar and arrange your schedules and make whatever it is into a "special event." You will be forever proud you did.

My mother had a knack for baking kolaches (a Czech pastry) better than anyone we knew. For years at family gatherings I would hear the grandchildren say, "Grandma, I wish you would teach me to make kolaches." She usually replied, "Yes, we should do that sometime," and years went by without our baking lesson. But one time we had the wisdom to get out a calendar and actually set a date to gather for kolach baking lessons. The deal was: each person who wanted to learn would come prepared with the ingredients to make one batch of kolaches. Mom would work from beginning to end with each one. We could all help along the way, but basically each person would be responsible for every step of their batch, and Mom would tutor each one individually. That's what we did. Mom patiently taught all day long.

When actual baking time came, the fabulous aroma of home-baked goods filled the neighborhood. We hung around the kitchen to watch the golden gems emerge from the oven—"oo-oo-ing," and "ahh-ahh-ing," tasting, and bursting our buttons with pride. We took photos all day long and sat before the loaded dining room table for a group picture with our sum total treasure when the day was done. Mom glowed with pride over both her students and the mass of baked goods. A wonderful "special event." The pictures hung on her wall for years so she could show and tell others, and the memories still last among us all.

Many people are in similar situations: unless they set a specific time to learn special skills and arts, those treasures will be lost and later lamented. Our ethnic backgrounds and cultural heritages are filled with ideas for such special events. Many cultures have unique foods, songs, chants, religious rites, poems, dances, prayers, and costumes associated with their celebrations. Have some fun creating special events around unique expressions to enjoy for their moments and pass on to the generations. *Now* is the best time to schedule a time and make a "special event" out of teaching and learning those specialties. Make the moments count!

Holidays

The way we celebrate holidays depends on many factors such as our ethnic heritage, the region of the country in which we live, our religious beliefs, the number, proximity, and relationship of family members, availability of friends, our financial resources, our health, and our interests. Holiday celebrations are often unique expressions of who we are and what is important to us. We need to pay attention to that uniqueness and celebrate it in spite of illness, disability, or even impending death. Holiday celebrations do not have to be elaborate, traditional, or people-filled in order to satisfy what is important to us. Very simple acknowledgment of the holiday can be as meaningful as an elaborate celebration. The caregiving process will add to the challenge of how we celebrate, but there will be opportunities to make the moments count. Holiday moments often become crystallized and are remembered days, months, and years after they happened.

Honey

Honey's son Greg and daughter-in-law Janice were caring for her following a diagnosis of a rapidly progressing brain tumor. Two of Honey's daughters and their families visited occasionally, but they expected to be away for the Christmas holiday. In past years, all had gathered at "Grandma's House," an apartment with a large recreation room just down the hall which they used for family gatherings. But so many things were different this year: "Grandma's House" didn't even exist anymore, because Honey had moved in with Greg and Janice; the other two families wouldn't be in the area at holiday time; and Honey was not her old self—although she had her good days, who could tell how she would be by Christmas? Honey and several other family members dreaded the holiday season. Greg and Janice had many conversations about what to do; Honey voiced her concerns, too. She thought they should just forget about Christmas this year.

But Greg had an idea two weeks before Thanksgiving. Since the whole family was planning to gather at Greg and Janice's home for Thanksgiving dinner, why couldn't they all celebrate both holidays at the same time? There was no need to forget about either one. Greg brought his idea to Janice and Honey, and they called other family members together and planned the dual holiday celebration. It turned into an adventure.

On Thanksgiving Day, all gathered and shared turkey dinner as always, except this time it was at Greg and Janice's home instead of at "Grandma's House." Each family brought their usual contribution to the dinner, and it was great. But it was what happened *after* dinner that was unique for this family.

After the dishes were washed and back in their places, Janice brought out the Christmas tree and boxes of lights and decorations. The group worked together to assemble the artificial tree, getting all the branches just right, and positioned it in its traditional place in the room—right in front of the living room window. Some unwrapped the ornaments and carefully placed them on the tree; others found decorations for windows, doors, and mantle and fit them into their niches. Honey supervised this whole "operation" from the living room sofa, suggesting the lights go here or an ornament go there. Janice put on a tape of Christmas music and some sang along. By late afternoon the place looked like Christmas and the group definitely was in the Christmas spirit.

On Thanksgiving Day in years past, the family tradition was to exchange names to determine who would give a gift to whom on Christmas Eve. Since there wasn't time for that this year, Greg had asked the group in phone conversations if he could expedite the process by writing everyone's name on a slip of paper, put them all in a hat and pull the names for everyone, then send them in the mail. All had agreed, so that's what he did. They had sufficient time to prepare the gifts and bring them along on Thanksgiving Day. So, when the Christmas atmosphere was in place, everyone sat down to exchange gifts in their usual Christmas tradition. It was enjoyable as always, but more moving this year. With Honey's health as it was, everyone seemed aware of the importance of these moments; this could be their last Christmas together.

When the gift giving was over, they sang a few Christmas carols as always and then brought out foods they usually served on Christmas Eve. By the time supper was over, it was clear that this family had, indeed, celebrated Christmas. And, oh, how pleased they were to tell their story to friends and relatives who gathered just three months later for Honey's funeral. It had been a unique holiday celebration for everyone, including Honey. They were proud they had celebrated while they all were able. By Christmas Honey spoke very little and slept a great deal of the time. Had they not celebrated Christmas on Thanksgiving Day, they would have missed their most memorable Christmas ever.

Just as Honey and her family had certain ways of celebrating, you and the person in your care have your own important holidays with your own specialties. Make adjustments in holidays and traditions, changing what you must and keeping what you can. If you are a family caregiver, you will be familiar with your family traditions. On the other hand, if you are a volunteer or in-home worker or professional, it will be up to you to find meaningful ways to celebrate holidays. Honey and her family kept most of their Christmas traditions but celebrated on a different day. It worked for them. Finding out what will work for you will take thought and perhaps several discussions with the others involved.

Your family, co-workers, or even your care receiver may not be as cooperative as the family members in Honey's story, who responded eagerly to Greg's suggestions. The people in your life may have ideas that conflict with yours or they may not want to be involved at all. Work with what you have and do the best you can. Keep your goals in mind rather than become enmeshed in uncooperative relationships or matters you cannot resolve. The goal is simply to make the holiday special—some way—and enjoy it. If it seems best to celebrate alone with the person, then enjoy that. Everything may not come out feeling like it took place in a storybook. That's okay. Make the moments count however you can. And, when the holiday is over, if things didn't work out as you had hoped, move on and look forward to something else rather than mentally rehashing what went wrong. You won't be able to change it anyway, so give yourself a break by looking forward rather than backward.

Celebrate all along the way; don't wait until it is "the last time." In the case of Honey we see a family gathering to celebrate knowing this might be their last holiday together. The person in your care may or may not be facing impending death, but when we think about it, we are *all* facing impending death. Each time we celebrate anything, it could be the "last time" for any of us. What a good reason to make the most of every opportunity to gather for important occasions and enjoy the company of those we love. If those we love are not available, holidays give us a good excuse to enjoy ourselves and life in the ways we can, while we can.

Arthur

Arthur's age and frailty necessitated several hours of assistance from home-health aides each week. He had lived alone since his wife died a year ago. She and Arthur had no children. Lois was a neighbor who realized that Arthur spent many hours alone, so she took on the role of being a volunteer visitor one afternoon each week. When February rolled around, Lois found Arthur more and more depressed. As she visited with him, he confided that he hoped he died before Valentine's Day because that time was hard since his wife died. Lois probed further into that subject and discovered that Arthur and his wife were married on Valentine's Day and always celebrated their anniversary by baking and sharing cookies. Lois remembered receiving some of their cookies in the past—they often shared them with neighbors, friends, and service people such as the mail carrier, neighborhood butcher and grocer. That was their favorite anniversary tradition.

As Lois thought about it, she decided that she and Arthur could bake Valentine cookies together and share them with neighbors just as Arthur and his wife had done in the past. Although Arthur did not feel very lively most days when Lois was there, he seemed more alert when he had something to occupy his mind and something to look forward to. Lois thought it was worth a try to find out more about the Valentine's Day traditions Arthur was used to and see how they could bring cookie baking into reality.

Lois used the "holidays" portion of the Checklist of Leisure Favorites to coax holiday-related information from Arthur. (Perhaps you will find it useful as well.) When Lois talked about holidays, Arthur was reluctant to share his memories. But as they discussed the Checklist, Lois nudged Arthur's memory into reminiscing about favorite holidays past. These discussions themselves were satisfying to Arthur. He seemed to find consolation in the good times he and his wife shared, and that brought a smile to his face.

As Lois brought up the idea of baking the Valentine cookies they used to share with neighbors, Arthur agreed to show Lois where to find the recipe for their sugar cookies and gave her orders about ingredients to purchase. Over the following two or three weeks, they set times to bake and decorate cookies and prepared them for neighbors. Although Arthur did not always feel up to it as planned and his participation was limited, they did manage to make and decorate two batches of cookies, and Arthur decided who should receive them. Lois packed the cookies carefully on small foil-covered trays, according to Arthur's directions. He signed cards that Lois brought over and tucked them into the packages, which Lois then delivered, in the name of Arthur, to neighbors and service friends. The best part came when they called Arthur or stopped by or sent cards to express their delight. The cookies were Arthur's means of staying connected to neighbors, friends, and the holiday. Lois realized that after they started baking the cookies, Arthur didn't talk much about wanting to die before Valentine's Day. He still was able to do something for someone else, in spite of his current condition. Both Lois and Arthur talked about baking those cookies long after that day.

Lois was able to find a way to modify cookie baking so Arthur could continue what had been an important tradition to him and his wife. Lois was wise to see how important this was to Arthur and then find a way to keep the tradition alive for him. Try to continue traditions if at all possible, being realistic about what health, stamina, or finances may allow at the present time. Most people have experienced some holiday traditions such as special foods, decorations, prayers or poems said on special occasions, or favorite people invited for the day. Be creative. Find substitutes if necessary; and if you aren't sure if a person has traditions, you can start new ones. Make it the "Best Ever Thanksgiving Box Cake" or a "Peanut Butter and Jelly Sandwich Birthday Party"—or whatever creative idea fits the situation.

A friend of mine who was feeling blue because she didn't get a birthday cake on her birthday called the grocery store to deliver two cupcakes along with her other groceries. Then, she stuck a candle in each and invited a friend from across her apartment hall to come in for a few minutes to enjoy her birthday cake. They laughed about it then and for many days after. It was a memorable birthday.

Sometimes, reminiscing about what holidays used to be can add to the fun if you take the positive side and smile about the memories rather than complain that it's not like it used to be. Be aware that reminiscing about past holidays might bring tears too, but direct those tears toward gratitude for the good times, and then do something to connect to those good times *now* through the traditions—whether they are cookies, songs, prayers, decorations, or people.

Often holidays are considered to be "family" days, and yet blood-family members are not always available to participate in holiday celebrations. It may be important to extend the idea of "family" to include the meaningful people who *are* available. I believe the idea of "family" needs to be extended, especially at holiday times. When there are few or no blood relatives to enjoy as family, create "family" by inviting others to fill that role. There may be others who are in the same position without "family"—acquaintances you feel can be supportive and willing to enjoy celebrating in nontraditional ways.

Outings

Here we will consider an "outing" any experience that broadens a person's world. We can broaden a person's horizon of the world in simple ways such as sitting a while in a room different from the usual routine; opening the drape and resting near the window in the sunshine; walking on the deck, patio, or balcony; or getting to the backyard for some fresh air and a walk on the grass. Sunshine, birds, trees, flowers, fresh air bring simple joys and healing feelings. Sometimes "armchair travel" provides a satisfying *vicarious* outing. Consider watching videos showing interesting places such as national parks, other states or countries, animals in a park or zoo, flowers and plants, museums and art exhibits. Family members or friends may come by to show slides of their trips to interesting places or share photos of places visited. Even travel magazines, brochures, and entertainment guides can give the sense of broadening a person's horizon.

Then, of course, there are the outings that take you and your care receiver beyond the home or caregiving setting. Depending on health and a variety of other circumstances, an outing may be easy or difficult to manage. Many caregivers are intimidated by the idea of taking someone out of the routine, protected environment. Fears of all kinds come up, such as the following:

⇨ How will I manage the movement, the transportation?
⇨ How far can we go?
⇨ How long can we be out?
⇨ How much help is needed?
⇨ Will people stare?
⇨ How will we manage the restroom?

Of all the concerns listed above, it seems that managing restroom needs causes the most concern among caregivers. Of course, it will always be easier to manage restroom needs, as well as other needs, if you have helpers along with you on the outing. If those helpers are familiar with the person's routines they will be more valuable than if you must familiarize them all along the way. If you or your helper are of the same gender as the person who needs care, you avoid at least one question of how to manage in the restroom. But sometimes, when a restroom need simply must be met, our choices are limited to "what works." I have found passersby to be quite helpful when asked to "stand guard" while I assist a man in the ladies' or if I need to enter the men's room with a man who needs assistance. Another option is to ask a manager or staff member of the facility to provide a solution to your need, perhaps providing access to an employees' facility or a private accommodation. It is concerns of this kind that often take the leisure out of a leisure outing!

No matter which questions come up, it will be important to think through all the details before venturing out. To save yourself a great deal of worry and wonder, it is wise to check out your destination before you get there. If you wonder whether or not there is enough space or light or an accessible entrance or helpful staff, pay a visit before the day of the outing. Sometimes, even when a facility is designated as accessible, it is difficult to negotiate ramps or elevators when you are managing the situation alone. Pay a visit, examine the place, and see how it feels. You can be comfortable, then, with all the details and save yourself from worry and unexpected difficulties at the time of the actual outing with your care receiver. Overall, it is helpful to keep outings simple.

Marshall

Doug made arrangements to spend Sundays with Marshall, whose frailty due to age now required that someone be with him most of the time. Other family members and home care workers shared responsibilities on the weekdays. Marshall had enjoyed his own home for over fifty years and wanted to stay just where he was. Doug encouraged him to go outside whenever the Sunday's weather permitted. Doug maneuvered the wheelchair into the yard so Marshall could see the street and watch the traffic go by.

Because Marshall enjoyed the outdoors so much, Doug was tempted to take Marshall to the zoo, to a shopping mall, or to visit a few relatives. But, luckily, his wisdom snapped into action. Marshall tired easily, and his pain and weakness made for a short attention span. So Doug decided that a drive to the ice cream shop would be enough. Marshall still could eat and enjoy ice cream, and he was able to get in and out of the car, so they went for the drive. Doug hopped out for ice cream cones, brought one to Marshall, and watched his face light up. They sat in the car and ate ice cream until it was gone, and then drove back home, looking at the sights along the way. It had been a great outing.

When it comes to outings, "less" is often "more." In other words, for the most enjoyment, keep outings simple. Doug seemed to know that, and Marshall's response to simply going out for an ice cream cone proved that Doug was right. Remember that after many hours or days or weeks inside, even a walk or wheelchair ride to the backyard can feel like a big deal, and a ride to an ice cream store may be a major event. Just because you would like to see someone get to this place or that event does not mean it will be a pleasant outing. This is an area where you must take note of your own needs and meet your needs independently from your care receiver. He or she might go along with an elaborate plan that you propose just to make *you* happy. Be sure the need, the person's interest, the health, and the motivation are all in line, and that the outing is suitable to the person before venturing out.

Also, keep outings realistic. Think through the details involved:

➪ How much energy will such a trip require in relation to energy available?

➪ How much help is needed in relation to what is available?

➪ Who is available to help? Will the assistants be volunteer or paid staff?

➪ How much money may be required in relation to money available?

➪ Can you manage the transportation or will you need help?

➪ What will happen if your care receiver needs to go to the restroom? (See discussion under "Outings," above.)

Be sure to plan according to the individual's interests. Find that "hot button" to know what will motivate someone to be willing to change the routine and venture out. Caregivers will find the "outings" portion of the Checklist of Leisure Favorites helpful in determining the outings that are realistic and desirable.

Mandy

Mandy, blind for the past year due to diabetes, lived with her daughter and family. When the family requested a friendly visitor for Mandy through their church, Doris decided she would enjoy befriending Mandy, and usually visited on Sunday mornings. After several months, Doris and Mandy became good friends. For her upcoming birthday, Doris wanted to do something special for Mandy, so she suggested they go out together for lunch. They set the day and time and selected a place.

When Doris arrived on the appointed day, Mandy was dressed and ready to go out, but she was very nervous and seemed quite upset. They continued with the plan, however, and arrived at the restaurant, where the situation got more and more complicated. Mandy was obviously embarrassed about her inability to read the menu; Doris kept reassuring her, but that didn't help. So Doris ordered something for both of them, and when the food arrived, Mandy was overly careful about every move; she was nervous and shaky and ultimately unable to enjoy what was meant to be a festive outing.

Doris learned a great deal from Mandy that day. She learned that what was special to her was not necessarily special to Mandy. She realized she was making Mandy's birthday special for herself and not necessarily for the honoree. Doris had not thought through everything involved in this celebration. Going out for lunch might have been a treat for Doris, but to Mandy, who was still adjusting to her blindness, it was a complicated, embarrassing ordeal. Mandy was too gracious to decline the invitation, wanting desperately to please her friend. Doris learned that they could have more fun making the day special at home. She decided that next time she would bring a bowl of fruit, and they could enjoy each other's company over fruit and tea on the deck. A much better outing! Be sure the outing suits the individual's wishes, interests, and abilities. Be sure to match the outing to the person.

In addition, take some time to prepare for the outing beforehand. This is not a time for the element of surprise. Discuss with the person things like what to expect, what to do, where you will be going, how long you plan to be there, what he or she would like to do there, and so on. Lay out plans and expectations clearly beforehand, so everyone involved can relax and enjoy a leisurely experience.

Fulfilling Unmet Dreams

As you and your care recipient reminisce about past good times, those memories may bring up a desire to do something just one more time, or they may be a reminder of a particular interest not yet pursued. An unmet dream may be simple or complex, depending on the person. You may be able to assist in fulfilling the dream—or at least a portion of it.

Garrett

Garrett loved baseball. All his life he enjoyed watching it on TV and listening to baseball games on radio, and generally he made it to a few home games during the season. Now he was fifty-eight and had leukemia, but baseball was still something he enjoyed. His condition required several hospitalizations alternated by periods when he could be at home in spite of severe weakness. Nino volunteered Monday evenings to give Garrett's wife some time off.

One Monday evening, while listening to the baseball game, Garrett told Nino that he wanted to get to one more game—not just listen to it, but go to the stadium just one more time. Nino thought about that and later talked to Garrett's wife, Lillian, to see if such a trip was possible. They agreed that it would be a big risk to get him to the stadium, but it would be a terrific idea. So they sat down with Garrett to think through everything involved. They did some strategizing.

Lillian admitted she would be concerned about taking a trip like that without some extra help. But she and Garrett thought they could hire an aide or a nurse from a home care agency to go along to help manage any critical situations that came up. The details seemed to be worked out, so Garrett decided on the day for the outing and on the game he wanted to see. Then, all they had to do was hope he would feel up to it when the time came, which he did. It turned out to be a great event. It didn't matter that the home team lost the game. They were all pleased to have taken the risk of helping Garrett fulfill one more dream.

Nino listened carefully to Garrett and heard him talk about his dream. Sometimes people "slip in" very important messages like that into casual conversations. If you really listen to what people say, sometimes you can hear them telling you their dreams. They often give you that information informally, and unless you are listening, it may pass you by. As you discuss the Checklist of Leisure Favorites with the person in your care, there will be many opportunities to listen for leisure interests, hobbies, or the dreams a person yearns to accomplish while still able. Take those comments seriously and consider the possibility of pursuing them if at all possible. If such ideas are indeed unrealistic, they may at least be the subject of conversation, even if they cannot become reality.

It may be necessary to seek help to meet the needs, just as we saw Nino consulting with Garrett's wife about how they could work together to meet the dream. If the dream entails unusual circumstances, discuss the plan with significant others. Think through all the details for safety and efficiency. There may be need for special transportation, nursing assistance, volunteers, special food accommodations, special lighting, seating, or sign interpretation. Look into all needs well in advance to prevent disappointment.

Vacationing

Christina

At age eighty-five Christina lived with her daughter Michele and son-in-law Les due to her poor mobility and health needs. She walked only short distances with difficulty and needed help with bathing and personal care. She used a cane regularly and a wheelchair when she went out. Michele and Les's large home gave her space and independence, and Michele and Les provided the supervision she needed.

The three of them plus Christina's son Fred were in the habit of taking vacations together. They enjoyed each other's company, liked to travel, and had taken a number of road trips. Christina was a good rider, able to sit comfortably in the back seat for long periods. She enjoyed seeing the scenery and equally enjoyed napping when tired. With frequent stops along the way, the four of them traveled well together. This year, Michele, Les, and Fred wanted to take Christina to Washington, D.C.—a trip she had dreamed of for years. Her dream was to see the changing of the guard at Arlington Cemetery and visit the national monuments.

But Christina objected to the idea. "I need too much help now. I would just be in the way," she kept saying. "You go and have a good time. I'll be all right here." Her "kids" thought she was well enough to make the trip although she would need a wheelchair and attention to her personal needs. But since they were in the habit of meeting those needs at home anyway, why couldn't they work together and manage the trip? They saw this as their last chance to take a major trip with their mom and make her dream come true. They set out to gather information.

They talked to a travel agent who informed them that the National Park Service in Washington provides an accessible van called the Tour Mobile with space for two wheelchairs, a lift, a driver, and a narrator to take persons with disability and their families to the national monuments. The fee is the same rate paid by other visitors who use the tourist shuttle service to and from the national monuments. With a call to the National Park Service they could make a reservation for the van on the specific day or days they would be there. They also looked ahead to their travel route and called motels to see if their accessible rooms would accommodate Christina, who could not climb into a bathtub without grab bars. Walk-in showers were best, but few motels or hotels had that facility. They did find enough accommodations to serve their needs, however, including a hotel in Washington close to the national sites.

After gathering information and planning how they would manage Christina's care, figuring out how they could pack her wheelchair on top of other gear in the trunk of the car, and promising each other to work as a team, they again presented the idea to Christina. "I'll think about it," she said. Several discussions followed. The "kids" continued to present all the reasons why the trip would be a good time for them all and reminded Christina that she always hoped and dreamed of seeing Washington, D.C. She, on the other hand, continued to present her case of not wanting to be a burden. Finally Les joked with her and said, "Besides, we want you to go because we really need your handicap parking permit!" Christina laughed and said, "Well, all right, then, let's go." Over the next weeks, they shared planning sessions and looked forward to their dream coming true. They considered details about Christina's care, necessary supplies, medications, schedules, and timing to prevent fatigue, and planned their strategies to make this trip work. They confirmed reservations, double checked information, marked maps, and packed lightly to leave room for the wheelchair.

Finally they set out for their adventure. Most motels along the way did meet Christina's needs, but sometimes she bathed at the sink because the tub was too high for her to get into or did not have grab bars. They arrived in Washington in the late afternoon, on schedule, and found that their hotel gave them a view of the Capitol. Christina looked out that window often. They spent the evening venturing out to eat and planning their upcoming routes on city maps. Since the accessible van traveled only on national park ground, they planned their alternate travel strategies. They knew they would need cab service or would have to push Christina for twelve or fourteen blocks at a time to reach their destinations. As it turned out, they did both in the course of the trip.

The next morning they took a cab to meet the National Park Service van, which they shared that day with another family whose father used a wheelchair. When the driver asked Christina, "Where to?", she said, "Arlington Cemetery to see the changing of the guard." From then on she had her list of places to see, and the driver took Christina and the family to each place, wheeled her to the destination, and made plans to pick them up when they wished. (The other family was accommodated in the same way—each family seeing a site while the other was transported.) The narrator used a microphone and gave tour information along the routes, and she called ahead for special accessible tours of the White House and the Capitol. Christina and the family were extremely impressed and grateful for all the friendly, skilled, accommodating services. In three days Christina saw all the places she had watched on the news and had hoped to see in person. Her dream vacation really did come true.

With good planning and plenty of help, even large dreams can be met. Reaching Christina's dream to see the nation's capital took considerable planning, mental and physical effort, personal and financial resources, her own willing spirit, and the teamwork of family and service personnel. Yet it *was* possible. Although there were moments of apprehension, everyone involved enjoyed the preparations, the actual experience, and fabulous memories for years to come. It was an event not only hoped for but actually scheduled and accomplished.

Your care receiver may or may not have vacation interests or dreams of this dimension, but even in the caregiving situation, it is possible to venture out and take large risks if all conditions can be worked out. Travel agencies have agents prepared to work with airlines, bus and train companies, hotels and motels, parks and attractions to accommodate the needs of persons with disability. Ask for the help and special accommodations you need. If Christina's family had not asked, they would not have discovered the Tour Mobile—accessible van service—available through the National Park Service (see the Related Resources section of this book). A librarian may also help you find travel directories of accessible hiking trails, state and national parks, hotels and motels. Local park and recreation personnel or therapeutic recreation specialists may be able to help you find information you need. If there is a dream to be met, be persistent about putting together "all the pieces of the puzzle" to make it happen. Be sure you have the assistance you need from family, friends, volunteers, or paid health-care workers to support the venture so everyone can enjoy the experience without burden or regret. And speaking of regret—take the trips and the outings, plan the special events, visits, and holiday celebrations while you can, before the time passes for those special moments, and you go on wishing you had done this or that. We only have the present moments. Make them count.

Summary

A wide range of leisure activities provide opportunity to build and maintain contacts with family, friends, the community, pets, plants, and our world in general. In the caregiving process, connections with others add to health and happiness whether it is through simple visiting or special events. Holidays and outings as well as very ordinary events become "special" when they are leisure experiences uniquely linked to values and beliefs. Special events provide an opportunity to celebrate our unique selves, including ethnic backgrounds, cultural heritages, relationships, religious beliefs, accomplishments, hopes and dreams.

Ideas for Staying in Touch with People and Other Living Things

⇨ Invite a friend or neighbor into the home
⇨ Visit friends, neighbors, or family members in their homes
⇨ Reminisce and tell stories with others
⇨ Play cards or table games with others
⇨ Go out for a small treat with a friend or family member
⇨ Go out for lunch with a friend, neighbor, or family member
⇨ Go out for a walk with a friend, neighbor, or family member
⇨ Visit a flower shop or garden nursery
⇨ Visit a pet store
⇨ Visit a zoo, park, or nature center
⇨ Watch people at a park or mall
⇨ Make contacts with special interest clubs and organizations
⇨ Stay in contact with members of former clubs and organizations

⇨ Keep the visits short and sweet
⇨ Plan simple activities to keep the visit interesting
⇨ Involve the person needing care in preparing for visits
⇨ Use the Checklist of Leisure Favorites to find social interests and needs

Ideas Regarding Holidays

⇨ Do what you can to keep holidays special
⇨ Follow traditions already in place
⇨ Create your own new traditions
⇨ Invite new people to replace "family" if necessary
⇨ Take the initiative to be creative in celebrating holidays

Ideas for Outings

⇨ Sit or lie in a room different from the usual routine
⇨ Sit near the window or on the deck in the sunshine
⇨ Go for a walk in the yard; pick some flowers (dandelions will do!)
⇨ Go to an ice cream store
⇨ Go for a car ride or a bus ride
⇨ Visit the home of a family member or friend
⇨ Go out for a meal or snack (drive through if that works best)
⇨ Go to church, temple, or synagogue
⇨ Go to sporting events
⇨ Go to a movie, concert, or play
⇨ Go shopping; go to the park
⇨ Go on a day trip, weekend trip, or a vacation
⇨ Do armchair travel: take a vicarious trip by way of videotapes, photos, books, visits from others with photos or slides from a trip
⇨ Keep outings simple and realistic; think through all aspects of the outing before leaving; check out facilities and accessibility prior to the outing
⇨ Plan according to the care recipient's condition, abilities, disabilities and interests
⇨ Try to fulfill unmet dreams

CHAPTER SEVEN

Spiritual Activity

BENEFITS
Spiritual activities make it possible to be in touch with one's Higher Power, express personal beliefs and values, collect thoughts, meditate, contemplate life and death, manage stress, appreciate beauty and life, and feel uplifted, motivated, inspired.

Many leisure experiences touch the human spirit and bring uplifting feelings to the person who enjoys them. These spiritual experiences are important to us as human beings as a way to find meaning in life. Spirituality, in the caregiving process as during other times of life, can be expressed through enjoyable activities. In this chapter I will discuss the following:

☆ Ideas for expressing the spiritual self through religion, nature, inspirational experiences, and a variety of other uplifting activities
☆ Stories that give examples of diversity in spiritual expression
☆ Spiritual and religious activity as leisure experience

Spiritual *Is a Broad Term*

Spirituality relates to the human spirit and meaningful expressions such as contemplation, religion, our philosophy of life, and our values. How people express their "inner spirit" varies from one person to another. For some people their spiritual activities are the same as their religious activities. For others, religion is not part of their spiritual ex-

perience. Instead, they find inspiration from a variety of other activities, many of which will be discussed in this chapter. In both cases,
however, people are able to express their spiritual selves and find the
peace of mind they seek. *Spiritual*, then, is a term that may or may not
include religion, depending on the individual's choice of expression.
In many respects, spirituality is an umbrella under which religious activity fits.

There is growing attention to spirituality in health-care and professional circles. Researchers are finding positive links between spiritual
activity and healthful outcomes. In a 1996 article for *USA Today*, Barbara Reynolds reported that of three hundred studies on spirituality
in scientific journals, the National Institute for Healthcare Research
found nearly three-fourths showed religion to have a positive effect on
health. In November 1996 the *Mayo Clinic Health Letter* cited studies that
showed that prayer may have improved the recoveries of heart bypass
patients; that regular church attendance may have helped reduce hy-
pertension in elderly men; and that religious faith helped ease the
emotional anguish of people having a diagnosis of cancer. Three years
earlier, Larry Dossey published a book called *Healing Words: The Power of
Prayer and the Practice of Medicine*, in which he reports numerous studies
showing that prayer helped alleviate high blood pressure, anxiety, and
headaches and promoted the healing of wounds. In 1994 Drs. Hani
Raul Khouzam and Charles E. Smith along with social worker Bruce
Bisset reported on various studies that linked religious beliefs to positive impact in later life and improved morale; also, church attendance,
prayers, and scripture reading were linked to helping older people cope
with problems of adjustment. They also reported that repeating Bible
verses to hospitalized veterans with dementia reduced the veterans'
agitation. Research points to the importance of the spiritual domain
of human behavior in health and wellness, especially as it relates to
people in their later years.

Spiritual activity definitely fits into the realm of leisure and needs
to be explored both in daily activity and in research. For some people,
leisure activities such as wilderness camping, growing plants, or jogging
serve as their spiritual expressions. How you incorporate spirituality
into your care receiver's life will depend on his or her interests and
beliefs.

Expressing Spiritual Feelings

Matt

Zach arranged to spend Saturday afternoons with Matt, who was in the progressive stages of AIDS. Some days Matt felt better than others, and Zach used those days to find how he could help him cope during both the good and bad days. Zach realized that he didn't know Matt very well, so he decided to use the "spiritual activity" portion of the Checklist of Leisure Favorites to find out what might bring Matt comfort during their Saturdays together. Completing the Checklist helped both of them find out how Matt could pursue an avenue of spiritual expression.

Zach noticed a variety of materials in Matt's apartment which evidently helped him express his spirituality. He had books with lovely nature photos, books of short stories and poetry, motivational tapes, audiotapes of nature sounds, tapes of favorite music, and several videos of national parks. Zach had a great idea. He knew that inspirational materials can help divert attention from pain and fatigue, so he helped Matt set up the tape player next to Matt's bed where he spent a good deal of time now, and where he could listen to his tapes in comfort. Zach asked Matt which tapes he most enjoyed and then stacked several on his nightstand where he could easily reach them. Matt remembered how much he enjoyed watching the videos of national parks and agreed that he might watch one from time to time if they were handy—which, of course, Zach quickly arranged. With Matt's consent, Zach moved the TV and VCR into Matt's room so he didn't even have to move to the living room to watch a video.

A person can express spiritual feelings through a wide variety of activities. In this case, inspirational materials helped Matt be in touch with his spiritual self. The videotapes of national parks were his way to connect with nature now that he was confined indoors. Many audio- and videotapes of nature sights and sounds are available to rent in local libraries and to purchase in various stores. Beautiful scenes, pleasing sounds, soothing music all serve to uplift the spirit. Consider how you might obtain such inspirational resources. By asking friends or notifying family members of your need for these, you may acquire a variety of inspirational materials.

It will be important that you accept the spiritual expressions of others—whatever they are. Your particular styles of spiritual expression may be different from those of the other person. Be open to the individuality of this part of life. This is not a time to try to convert someone to your spiritual ways and beliefs. Rather, your part is to make available spiritual opportunities that are satisfying to the person in your care. Help him or her find simple, meaningful ways to express the spiritual self and feel uplifted.

Religious Activity

Everette

After months of battling colon cancer, Everette asked his wife Barbara, their daughters, and other family members to let him die at home rather than spend his last weeks in a hospital. Although the intensive tasks required to meet his wishes frightened Barbara, she thought she could do it with the help of extended family. As a team, Everette's mother, two brothers, and two sisters arranged their schedules as needed. As days wore on, their hours overlapped and lengthened. Everette's only comfortable position eventually was reclining in his living room easy chair, so all caregiving took place there. The family consulted with the medical staff, but overall they functioned on their own. They managed their own stress with brief outdoor walks, visits with friends, hugs, shooting baskets in a nearby gymnasium, reading poetry, talking and crying together, preparing family favorite foods, and praying.

Over the years the Catholic faith had been a strong element of their family life, and everyone engaged in Everette's last days found support in their beliefs. Family members prayed individually with Everette from time to time when he was awake; they prayed together at meals and in the evenings and during their night watches. Their parish priest not only stopped by to visit Everette and the family but offered to say Mass in the home, in the living room where Everette rested. This event proved to be especially meaningful to everyone. It was an experience that further solidified their spiritual and family ties.

Everette's two daughters, ages nine and eleven, were active participants in the family caregiving operations. They held their dad's hand while he rested, sat on his lap for short evening visits when he was awake, and showed him their school work and art pictures. In these moments Everette prepared his daughters for his death, told them how much he loved them, and reminisced with them about their lives together. On some days older family members took the girls to the park or a movie to break out of the home scene.

When the day of Everette's death came, family members had already done some of their mourning, and their family bonds were closer than ever. Not only had they met Everette's last wishes, but they had experienced a spiritual bonding with him and with each other.

Family researchers M. A. Lieberman and L. Fisher noted in 1995 that when family members care for one of their members who has an illness, it truly is a *family affair*. When a team effort among family members develops in the caregiving process, it is possible for the whole family to grow together, in spite of losing one member. The Catholic religion played a large role in the case of Everette, but the family relationships also provided part of the spiritual experience surrounding his death—for him and for the other members. That is not unusual. Joseph Dancy and Lorraine Wynn-Dancy have pointed out that sometimes warm and sympathetic human relationships serve our spiritual needs. Of course, not every member of every family will rally to meet a need, as happened in Everette's case. However, we can learn from the spiritual impact of the relationships we see here. As a caregiver, try to bring close to you meaningful people who can be your emotional and spiritual support. For your care receiver, there may be important persons to invite in to bring their spiritual comfort to him or her.

Religious rituals and practices help meet spiritual needs. Prayers and religious rites and services can be comforting and inspiring especially during times of illness and impending death. If you are a family caregiver, you are familiar with former religious practices, and this will make it easier to provide those comforting options. If you are a volunteer, in-home worker, or professional, finding out this information and making opportunities available for familiar rituals will be important. Ministers, rabbis, and other religious leaders are often willing to visit a person who is homebound and may even be able to conduct home services if asked.

Homebound people miss their church or synagogue and need visits from members of their congregations. "Prayer at home and watching religious programs on television do not always provide the kind of continuity needed to preserve . . . meaningful religious identity," gerontologist Sheldon Tobin noted in 1991. Tobin further pointed out that home visitation by faith congregations has, for centuries, been a primary means of ministering to those who are ill or disabled, and this continues today. If your care receiver wants to stay connected with the faith community, you can contact leaders or members of the congregation and ask for the desired home ministry. This will not be placing a burden on the congregation but rather be giving members opportunity to minister as they are called to do.

Children also can play important roles in caregiving and spiritual experience. Just as Everette's daughters were actively involved in his last days, other children deserve to be part of such family events. Everette's daughters' moments with their father were spiritual encounters that connected them to him then, and to the ongoing memory of him. The girls' visits were important leisure moments in their lives and his. Not every child, however, may want to be a part of the caregiving scene. Children can participate to the extent they are comfortable.

Hanna

Hanna, eighty-nine years old, was recovering from a hip injury and living in the home of her son and his family. Family members took turns caregiving and spending time with her. Jim, her son, knew how important literature, poetry, scripture, and prayer were to his mother throughout her life. Sometimes they prayed together, saying out loud some of the prayers they prayed in their family over the years. One evening, Jim asked Hanna if she would like him to read something to her. Her eyes lit up at the idea. She said some poetry would be nice or maybe some scripture. So Jim brought out a book of poetry and his Bible. After some visiting, Jim read several poems to Hanna. They discussed some special parts, but mostly Hanna just smiled. Sometimes they were just silent together, reveling in the meaning of what was read. Jim ended the visit with two of Hanna's favorite Psalms, and then she closed her eyes to rest. He left without further chatting. He did not want to break the spiritual mood created through the poetry and scripture.

Jim had the advantage of knowing his mother over his lifetime; because he was familiar with her favorite prayers and readings, he could easily find inspirational materials that were meaningful to her. If you are a family caregiver, you are more likely to know the traditions of the person in your care and how spiritual needs have been met in your family. A person's favorite ways of spiritual expression may change over time, though, and you may or may not be correct in what you think is meaningful. Even for a family member, it is useful to talk about and try to discover the real favorites, so that spiritual expression is easy.

Jim felt comfortable praying with Hanna because they knew the same prayers and had prayed together many times over the years. As a caregiver, you may or may not know your care receiver's prayers or spiritual habits. You may not even feel comfortable praying with the person, especially out loud. Besides family members, sometimes volunteer visitors from the person's church, temple, or synagogue are the best ones to initiate praying with the person. If you know the person well, however, or if he or she has indicated to you an interest in praying together, you might find this an especially meaningful thing to do. Many people learned prayers early in their lives, and those prayers are part of their long-term memory, which often remains intact for a long time in spite of illness, disability, or dementia. When that is the case, reciting prayers may come automatically, and saying prayers aloud may be one of the few things you can still do together.

It may be because Jim knew his mother so well that he was comfortable being silent with her. Sometimes it is difficult to just be quiet and let yourself or another person deeply experience a spiritual moment. Try to be comfortable with silence. You do not need to fill every minute with activity or talk. Quiet moments are necessary for a person to find and express the spiritual self. Nor do you need to keep someone busy during every waking hour. Silence is *not* nothing. It can be powerful and pleasurable. Just enjoy being at peace together in silence from time to time. Let the spiritual experience speak for itself. It is not necessary to talk about every spiritual experience. Because of the personal nature of this aspect of life, some people like to relish these moments internally. Be sensitive to the person's preference, and "just let it be" when that feels best.

Nature

Leandra

Following diagnosis of a rare cancer, Leandra, thirty-two, chose to go to the lake home of her grandparents after her cyclic intensive chemotherapy treatments. Her system reacted severely to each treatment, and she knew she needed spiritual support to endure each bout. She chose this place to be during the difficult times because of the close contact she could have with nature. All her life she had come here to sit on the lakeshore, watch birds on the steamy lake in the early mornings, catch butterflies, play with the dog and cat, relish the color in her grandmother's flower garden, and marvel at the sunsets. Now, when her grandparents invited her to rest and recover at their home, she knew it was the place to be.

Leandra's grandmother looked after her needs very well, preparing the few foods that she could eat and providing for her comfort as much as possible. But mostly Leandra needed what nature offered her here. When she felt up to it she sat in her "special place" on a lakeshore rock where she contemplated life and her possible death. She felt comforted here and a sort of healing took place deep inside. On the days she did not feel like being up, she still could see the lake, birds, flowers, trees, clouds, and sunsets from her window and feel close to nature. Porky the dog and Rusty the cat came to see her when she couldn't get out to be with them. Nature helped her find comfort in spite of her physical pain.

As you read about Leandra, perhaps you could visualize the lake scene and recall similar places that served your own spiritual needs. Having a "special place" is useful in times of both health and illness. A person's special place does not need to be exotic or far away. In fact, when your "special place" is near and easily accessible, you can get to it often rather than on special occasions only. It may be as handy as a favorite lawn chair in view of flowers, a walkway in a neighborhood park, a museum courtyard, a comfortable bench in an art gallery, your own orchard, a small creek on adjoining property, or a large "sitting rock" in the woods. Everyone needs a special place to rest, collect thoughts, and be in touch with the spirit within. An indoor space such as a favorite rocking chair, an art-filled room, or a comfortable chair by a sunny window may serve as your "special place" as well. The important thing is to *have* that place where you can go often and feel whole when you are there.

Nature offers spiritual experiences of comfort and healing. The ancient Greek and Roman cultures used beautiful gardens, courtyards, and scenic walks as healing settings for persons who were ill. A lake home with its natural beauty may not be available in your caregiving situation as it was for Leandra, but there are other ways to bring a person into contact with nature. Depending on your situation, consider these possibilities for a nature experience: sitting in the yard or on the porch or deck to see elements of nature, feel breezes and warm temperatures; walking or wheeling through a flower garden to smell fragrances and delight in the colors; walking or wheeling in a neighborhood park to absorb its beauty; visiting a zoo to be in touch with the animals; going fishing or camping; or watching stars at night either outside or through the window.

If someone is unable to get out of the house or even out of bed, you can bring elements of nature inside for close encounter. Try bringing in things such as sand from a beach and sift through it to find shells and pretty stones; seaweed and salt water to smell, touch, and reminisce over; stones, rocks, shells; weeds and wildflowers; flowers to smell and arrange in a vase to keep at the bedside or within view; butterflies and insects in a jar to watch and then release; colored feathers to feel and talk about; dried flowers, weeds, and colored leaves in the fall of the year. Watching fish in an aquarium may also be uplifting. Be creative and find interesting items that will provide opportunity to wonder at and appreciate nature's beauty.

Even without direct contact with nature, a person can envision real or imagined beautiful places and create a "special place" in the mind. The mental activity called imaging allows a person to transport in mind to a spiritual realm of experience. Therapeutic recreation professor David R. Austin explained in 1997 that "imagery" refers to using positive suggestions to create mental representations of things we know or can fantasize. Stress management exercises frequently use imagery to control thoughts and focus the mind on soothing scenes and feelings. If the person is able to follow the words and is interested in participating in imaging activity, the following words may be used as guides to an

uplifting experience. In his 1983 book *Leisure Wellness*, C. Forrest Mc-
Dowell suggested creating a "private place" for purposes of relaxation,
refreshment, and healing. Based on some of his ideas, I developed the
following exercise which you and your care receiver may find spiritu-
ally uplifting.

A "Special Place"

For a mental "visit to a special place," read, out loud, the following sentences *slowly*, in a gentle, comforting voice, allowing time to imagine
the suggested scenes.

1. Close your eyes; get comfortable; breathe in and out deeply,
    steadily.
2. Continue to breathe deeply, and in your mind's eye take yourself
    on a walk along a beautiful path.
3. Notice the beauty around you as you walk: lush green plants;
    beautiful, fragrant flowers; fresh running water; birds singing
    sweetly; blue sky and warm sunshine. Feel and experience every
    element nature has to offer.
4. This pathway takes you to a clearing where you find a very spe-
    cial, beautiful place. As you look around, you notice a comfortable
    resting place. You sit down, take a deep breath, and drink in the
    beauty around you.
5. Take special notice of the trees, the flowers, birds, gentle animals,
    sun, sky, water, warmth, and comfort. Enjoy the colors, fra-
    grances, sights, sounds, and good feelings here.
6. This is your special place. Here no one can find you. Here no one
    can harm you. Here you feel whole and refreshed. You can come
    here whenever you want to find beauty, peace, quiet, comfort,
    and rest.
7. Look around and take in the details of this special place. Picture
    it clearly in your mind so you can come here quickly and often if
    you wish.
8. Take time to rest in your special place. Enjoy the good feelings.
9. When you are ready, follow the beautiful path back to the room,
    knowing you can return in your mind to your special place when-
    ever you wish.

10. When you return, gently open your eyes, stretch, and relish the good feelings you brought with you from your special place.

Following this imaging activity, you may want to let the experience just "speak for itself"—it may even remain more "real" if you don't talk about it. It is possible that this activity, which is pleasant for most people, will be uncomfortable for some. As always, pay attention to your care receiver's responses. Only when he or she responds positively should the activity be continued or repeated.

Summary

Spiritual activity is an important area of leisure experience that includes religious activities as well as a wide variety of other means of expressing the spiritual self. In the caregiving process, both care receiver and caregiver can find uplifting moments individually and jointly through spiritual expression. Since spirituality can be expressed through religious as well as other means, accept the spiritual expressions of others—whatever they are. Be comfortable with silence, and let the spiritual experience "speak" for itself when that feels best.

Spiritual Activity Ideas

⇨ Read spiritual materials such as the Bible, the Koran, the Talmud, and other holy books, spiritual greeting cards, classics, poetry, inspirational stories, devotional books and calendars, art books
⇨ Pray; contemplate, and meditate
⇨ Attend religious services
⇨ Listen to tapes of services
⇨ Participate in socials at church, temple, or synagogue
⇨ Visit with minister, priest, rabbi, or other spiritual advisor
⇨ Listen to or watch religious services on radio and TV
⇨ Visit with people from church, temple, or synagogue
⇨ Contemplate and discuss life after death, values, meaningful life and death issues
⇨ Read and write poetry
⇨ Memorize inspirational quotations
⇨ Look at inspirational pictures: photos, posters, art books

⇨ Enjoy nature; visit inspirational places; spend time in a real or imagined special place
⇨ Wander through an art gallery, a crafts shop, or a natural history museum
⇨ Listen to comforting, inspirational music
⇨ Listen to inspirational audiotapes and tapes of nature sounds
⇨ Watch inspirational videotapes
⇨ Do yoga; do deep breathing
⇨ Keep a personal journal
⇨ Just be quiet

CHAPTER EIGHT

Planning for Meaningful Activity

Now that we have considered the full range of physical, intellectual, emotional and expressive, social, and spiritual activities, it is time to think about how to plan them into the caregiving days. In this chapter I will discuss the following:

☆ The importance of planning leisure activities
☆ Arranging schedules around a person's unique needs
☆ How to make the most of leisure activities
☆ Setting a simple leisure plan for every day
☆ Sample leisure plans
☆ Documenting and evaluating the leisure moments you share with your care recipient

Do you remember mornings when you hopped out of bed because you had something special on your calendar, something you had been waiting for? Maybe it was the first day of school, or a family vacation, or visiting a special friend. Now, and even more importantly *now*, when days are more difficult because of caregiving tasks and the illness, disability, or confinement of your care receiver, you both need something to look forward to, every single day.

For this to happen, you will need to make plans and follow through on them. Maybe some of the suggestions for leisure moments described in the previous chapters appealed to you, but they will remain *just ideas* unless you bring them into reality. Rather than saying, "Oh, we should do that sometime," actually plan and schedule a leisure moment into every day. The activity ideas in this book provide the basis for sharing meaningful moments that can become long-lasting, fond memories.

Arranging Schedules to Fit the Person

In Chapter 2 we discussed the importance of finding the leisure "hot buttons" that motivate a person to "get up and go" and participate in favorite activities. Just knowing what these hot buttons are won't make things happen, however. You need to apply that information to a *plan of action* and a *plan for enjoyment*. This kind of planning does not require long lists of supplies or equipment. It requires simply thinking about how to blend a little enjoyment into every day. You can start by setting a plan that follows the person's natural rhythms.

Ming

Ming, a woman with severe rheumatoid arthritis, has been cared for by her husband Li for many years. Her pain and stiffness prevent her from getting out of the house very often, and Li has become adept at assisting her. When Li was asked how he and Ming manage, he said: "We have a routine. That helps. She likes to sleep late and move slowly, I like to rise early and get going. So, I'm up early, go for my walk, go out for breakfast, and by mid-morning when I come back to the house, Ming's about ready to get up. That's when I help her with her daily routine. It all goes pretty well as long as I do things for her according to her schedule and not mine. She never did like to get up early, so I know enough to go by her inner clock. Ming likes to watch late movies on TV, too, but I like to retire early. I set up her room with the TV positioned so she can see it from her pillow. She has a remote control at her bedside that she can reach when she wants it. I sleep in the next room, and I go to bed when I like. She knows she can call me if she needs me. We both do best when we stick to our own schedules."

As a caregiver, you know that Li is giving good advice. Things just go better when we go along with people's natural schedules. Li claims that every day holds more than enough challenges without going against each other's inner clocks, so keeping his schedule while also going along with Ming's schedule has helped them both. The Checklist of

Leisure Favorites has a section on the daily schedule; it may help you to make the best arrangements for leisure activities in each day.

Making Plans for Each Day

When an activity is meaningful, and not just a time filler, we enjoy it before, during, and afterwards. The first phase—*looking forward*—is key to having something to get up for each day. The expectation itself is a worthwhile activity. The second step is *doing the activity*: the real event that we looked forward to, whether or not it lives up to our expectations. The third step is the follow-up—*recalling the activity*. This part can turn into the enjoyment of long-lasting fond memories, as well as interesting visual or audio records of what took place.

The follow-up is also key to the next plan. If the activity turned out to be satisfying, we look forward to doing it again; if it didn't, we are skeptical about planning it again and look for another choice. Make the most of every phase of activities. Enjoy the planning and the anticipation, enjoy the activity, and enjoy the follow-up; talk about what you did, put pictures in a scrapbook, or read through brochures or other literature related to the activity.

Conchita

After Conchita's stroke and return home from the hospital, her family requested a volunteer to spend some afternoons with her to provide relief for family caregivers. Marlis decided to help out. During her first volunteer visit, she made lunch for the two of them and washed the dishes. When the chores were done, they rested and watched TV, but as time went on, Marlis grew bored and apprehensive: What will they do all afternoon? It wasn't even snack time, and the afternoon was already long. Besides, Conchita was restless; her attention span didn't allow for watching much TV. Marlis knew she had to do some planning for each day, or both of them would find this arrangement difficult. Marlis decided to involve Conchita in preparing meals as much as possible, and to plan at least one other activity for every day, yet be flexible about the plans in case Conchita didn't feel up to it. She decided to set aside a little time during each visit to make some plans with Conchita—deciding what they could do together next time.

Setting an Activity Goal

Set an activity goal for every day so you both have something to look forward to. It may be something as simple as frosting a cake (or at least licking the spoon), looking through a kaleidoscope, or tinkering in the garage. The previous chapters detailed numerous physical, intellectual, emotional, social, and spiritual activities. Consider the type of activity the person most needs or wants. If possible, talk over with the person various ideas about what to do, when to do it, who to invite, what foods to serve, and so on. Planning *with* and not *for*, whenever possible, will enhance a sense of control and dignity. Together, look through this book for ideas. If you include something from each chapter into each week, you both will experience an interesting variety of activities that touch all the behavioral domains (as discussed in Chapter 2).

Looking forward makes the difference between living every day rather than just making it through the day. When there is something to look forward to, you have more to talk about and more motivation to make it through less pleasant tasks. For example, looking forward to sitting on the porch in the afternoon may make it worth the effort to get out of night clothes and dress in a shirt and slacks. While working through the dressing tasks, you can talk about the birds, sunshine, and shade trees to be enjoyed in the backyard later in the day. Or, looking forward to an after school visit from a neighborhood child may provide motivation to send an invitation or make a phone call to arrange the visit and then, on the appointed day, to work together to make a batch of marshmallow treats to share during the visit. All along the way, you can talk about the plan, the child, the good time you expect to enjoy. With such simple plans in the caregiving process, each day is unique and interesting in spite of the tasks that must be accomplished. Make plans, "talk up" the plans, put up signs and posters to remind everyone involved that there is something to look forward to.

Here are some sample daily goals to plan and post:

➪ Sit out on the porch and watch traffic, birds, people, clouds
➪ Play favorite card game or table game before supper
➪ Listen to Talking Books after nap time
➪ Sing along with a tape, CD, record, or the radio

⇨ Play the piano or other musical instrument (even a kazoo!)

⇨ Listen to favorite music album

⇨ Cut out pictures from magazines; make a collage

⇨ Read a book or story out loud; discuss the favorite parts

⇨ Make a snack together and enjoy eating it

⇨ While making lunch, take spices from the kitchen cupboard and identify them by their aromas

⇨ Make an after school treat for a neighbor child and invite her over

⇨ Organize shelf or drawer or box; reminisce and tell stories about the items inside

⇨ Put together a jig-saw puzzle; work on a word game or crossword puzzle

⇨ Check out the moon and stars, either outside or through the window with the lights out

⇨ Try a new flavor of tea with lunch

⇨ Watch a favorite video

⇨ Read humor from the *Reader's Digest* during the afternoon

⇨ Walk or wheel to the mailbox when the mail arrives

⇨ Write (perhaps through dictation) a letter to a friend or relative

⇨ Read "Dear Abby" and/or comic strips in the newspaper; discuss

⇨ Open the living room drapes and sit in the afternoon sun

⇨ Have a paper airplane contest

⇨ Try to learn a magic trick

⇨ Go out for an ice cream cone, or have one at home

⇨ Listen to a radio talk show and discuss the topic between yourselves

⇨ Look through old photos and tell stories about the events pictured

⇨ Make a craft or holiday decoration

⇨ Sit inside or outside and watch the birds early in the morning; set up a bird feeder if there isn't one

⇨ Look through a catalog and make a wish list

⇨ Look through travel brochures; tell stories about or plan a dream vacation

⇨ Look at maps of places to go or places enjoyed in the past

⇨ Take down clutter off a shelf; sort through items one at a time

⇨ Bring some roses (or other flowers) and *really* smell them

Planning Ahead

Whether you are planning a shared leisure moment with your care receiver, a leisure pursuit for the person alone, or a leisure break for yourself as caregiver, consider these factors:

What need do we want to fill?
Physical? Intellectual? Emotional? Social? Spiritual?
What would feel best right now? What is the need?

⇨ to get a little exercise?
⇨ to keep the mind active?
⇨ to divert attention from pain?
⇨ to get feelings out into the open?
⇨ to laugh?
⇨ to see other people?
⇨ to be of service and contribute to others in some way?
⇨ to be in touch with nature?
⇨ to be quiet within oneself?

Activities can fulfill a variety of needs. When we know what we want from activities, we can select the best activities to meet those needs.

What specific activity best fits the need right now? Match the physical, intellectual, emotional, social, and spiritual needs with activity ideas in the chapters of the book. Select an activity that will meet the need you want to fill—by thinking like this:

⇨ If the person has had little opportunity to be physically active lately, perhaps an activity that includes movement would be useful and enjoyable.
⇨ If some mental stimulation is needed now, check suitable activity options related to intellectual activity.
⇨ If your care recipient has had pent-up feelings lately, perhaps emotional activities would provide an avenue for expressing those feelings.
⇨ If loneliness is a problem, consider the possibility that social activities would help to make connections with others.

⇨ When there is a need to be alone with inner thoughts, suggest spiritual activities.

Also use the Checklist of Leisure Favorites to plan activities based on favorites. Involve your care recipient in planning activities as much as possible. When you plan together with those who will participate, each of you makes an investment in the planned activity and is more likely to participate when the time comes.

When can we do the selected activity? When you set a specific time for the activity, both you and the care recipient have something to look forward to and plan around. If you designate the time as "right after lunch" or "just before supper," this will be specific enough to make it happen. It is also more likely that you will actually accomplish the activity this way than if you just say, "Maybe we'll do that later." If possible, together discuss when you will do things such as go on a small shopping trip for toiletries, cut coupons from the paper, or read aloud the next chapter of a continuing story. This doesn't mean you have to be rigid about the plan, however.

How can we build flexibility into the plan? Always have an alternate plan in mind so you can adjust to changes in health, weather, and mood. Remember, *leisure* means "freedom from necessity." Being flexible will be important to keeping the leisure spirit of your plan. This means that even when you set a plan to enjoy an activity, the plan needs to remain free from added burden, guilt, or trouble. When sudden changes come up, keep the plan on hold until the next right moment. Or, make an adjustment to carry out some part of the activity rather than the whole. It is best to have several things in mind as contingency plans; these are things you can do when the person does respond and is interested in participating. But if you never have a plan in mind, those moments of possible enjoyment will come and go without making them count.

Sometimes things don't happen unless we have a written plan. It doesn't have to be elaborate. In fact, it can be as simple as four lines, like the following:

Our Plans

The activity:
The best place:

The best time:
Things to prepare beforehand:

Here are a few completed written plans that are examples of how you can plan:

Our Plans

The activity: put a puzzle together
The place: living room, at the card table
The best time: Monday P.M., after nap
Things to prepare beforehand: put up card table and chairs; find a
    favorite puzzle with no more than one hundred pieces

The activity: look through photo albums
The place: at kitchen table
The best time: Wednesday, after supper
Things to prepare beforehand: clear the table; bring out a few
    albums so George can choose favorite

The activity: go shopping for a shirt
The place: downtown mall
The best time: Thursday, after lunch and nap
Things to prepare beforehand: set out clothing; take money; clear
    trunk of car for wheelchair; call to check location of restrooms
    at the mall

The activity: write letter to Leo in Germany
The place: kitchen table
The best time: Friday afternoon
Things to prepare beforehand: find stationery, pen, stamps

The activity: make peach jam
The place: kitchen
The best time: afternoon, after George's nap
Things to prepare beforehand: peaches, jars, sugar, pectin, bowls,
    spoons

The activity: Sunday visit from church visitor

The place: living room
The best time: 10:00 A.M.
Things to prepare beforehand: be sure George is dressed in time
    for visit

Making the Most of the Plan

You can make the most of the plan and the activity in these ways:

Before the activity

➪ Set a plan that is clear and realistic. Plan what you will do, when
   you will do it, and think through what materials you will need.
➪ Be a salesperson for the upcoming activity. You can promote
   the plan, or "talk it up," while you do other things together, reminisce about previous activities, or extend a special invitation to
   participate.
➪ Put up a sign naming the activity and noting when it is to take
   place. A piece of notebook paper will do. Decorate it or not, according to personal preferences; sometimes drawing an activity-
   appropriate picture, like a cookie for a planned baking activity, can
   add a little fun. Post the note on the refrigerator or in the bedroom or on the bathroom mirror or some other prominent place
   so everyone can see it and look forward to the experience.

During the activity

➪ Make the most of the moments when you do the activity. Remem-
   ber, the *enjoyment* during the activity is what counts.
➪ Do everything you can to build self-esteem and good feelings.
   Help the participant (and yourself) have a good time.
➪ Relax and enjoy whatever happens even if it is not exactly what
   you had planned.

After the activity

➪ Relive the event by remembering together what took place.
➪ Bring up the special or humorous moments as a topic of conversation, as a distraction from pain, or as means of looking forward to
   another activity.

⇨ If an activity did not go well, use what you learned to make another plan, and try to improve the outcome.

⇨ If you keep a record of what took place, you will have information to remind you of what went well and what didn't, so you can plan well for next time. (Sample records appear later in this chapter.)

It's helpful to see each activity as a process rather than as an end in itself (process has the "before, during, and after" elements). Don't worry about everything being perfect or coming out just as planned. Rather, relax, and let one activity lead to another. Once you begin adding simple leisure experiences to caregiving, you will find it easier and easier to plan them and make them beneficial for your care receiver—and for you, too. Let your shared enjoyment lead you, and try not to be concerned about whether or not others think the activity was a success. Judge success by what happens all along the way, not only by what the end product looks like. If you are baking cookies together, try to enjoy every step, from sifting the flour through mixing and baking, all the way to tasting. If the final product doesn't look like something at a bake-off contest, it doesn't matter, because the *process* counts, too. How much you giggled when you stuck flour on each other's noses and how you enjoyed the aroma of the baking cookies are part of the process—and just as important as eating tasty cookies.

Keeping Records

When you keep track of how leisure activities go—whether or not they were eagerly looked forward to, whether they were fun and interesting, and whether they provided fond memories afterwards—you gather important information to use for ongoing planning. Your records will not only help you as you look ahead, but they may become the source of memories to enjoy in the future. There are many simple ways to keep track of the good times you share and many possible ways to record events and memories to keep them fresh for a short time or for years to come.

Keeping a log, diary, or journal of leisure-time activities may be one of the most familiar ways to keep track of what you do. You can note what happened when, where, with whom, and who enjoyed what.

Note, too, the activities that did not go well and what you would avoid or improve next time. Caregivers often keep a daily log of the care receiver's health conditions and responses; the leisure data can be added to show the full picture of current status and to pass on to other caregivers. I find that recording information under the following topics can give a good picture of what took place as well as give direction to the next activity plan:

Our Record

The activity:
The outcome:
Things to change next time:

Here are a few sample entries, kept in a simple lined notebook called *Our Record*:

The activity: 9/8/97: We worked on jigsaw puzzle this P.M. (George chose the rocket picture).
The outcome: We completed frame of puzzle; G. wants to finish tomorrow; he told stories about doing puzzles with his mother.
What to change next time: Try puzzle before lunch; maybe he'll be less tired.

The activity: 9/9/97: We finished the puzzle.
The outcome: Before lunch *was* a better time; George seemed surprised that we got it finished; he doesn't want to take it apart yet—we'll leave it on the card table in the living room a few days.
Things to change next time: Look for another 100-piece puzzle.

The activity: 9/10/97: George looked at pictures of trip to mountains for about 35 minutes.
The outcome: He laughed at his long hair and remembered some wildlife he had seen; the moose were his favorite.
Things to change next time: Nothing! Do it again soon.

The activity: 9/11/97: Shopped at mall for shirt.

The outcome: Found shirt at right price after much looking;
   George got tired and restless; stayed too long.
Things to change next time: Call stores before we go—to check
   styles and prices—to cut down on stops. (Restrooms are handy
   on the east side.) Stop for ice cream on the way home!

The activity: 9/12/97: Read Leo's last letter again; G. dictated and
   I wrote what he wanted to say to Leo.
The outcome: He had a hard time thinking of things to say, but we
   got a pretty good letter written. George misses Leo (so do I); we
   both cried a little.
Things to change next time: Nothing! Do it again.

The activity: 9/13/97: Made peach jam.
The outcome: It looks and tastes great! George read me the
   directions, and he did the stirring. He wants to give a jar to
   Gladys tomorrow.
Things to change next time: Scald and peel peaches before G. gets
   involved—so he doesn't get so tired.

The activity: 9/14/97: Sunday visit from Gladys (visitor from
   church).
The outcome: Gladys prayed with George, then visited. Lively
   visit—George told about making jam and gave a jar to Gladys.
   We ate jam on crackers together. Pretty good!
Things to change next time: Nothing! Gladys is a "bright spot" on
   Sunday.

There are many other ways to keep records of your activities besides keeping a log. Here are some suggestions:

⇨ Keep a poster on the wall if it is helpful for your care receiver and
   other people to see at a glance the activities you have enjoyed.
   You can use a marker to note what you did, where you went, and
   who participated.
⇨ Take snapshots of events as they happen; capture the smiles,

frowns, friendships, and feats. Post them with captions in a prominent place to enjoy and to show visitors. Use them to reminisce
and tell the stories over and over.

➪ Take video footage of events in progress; watch them again and
again.

➪ Make an audio- or videotape of an "interview" with someone discussing the good time you had collecting wildflowers, watching
porpoises, or riding in a horse-drawn carriage.

➪ Draw pictures of what you did and the way you each felt while
you did it. Line drawings can be expressive; artistic talent is *not* required for this one; it is about expressing feelings—whatever they
are, happy or sad or in between.

➪ Call a local newspaper to cover a planned activity. Or, write an
article for the local newspaper telling who did what when and
where and how much it was enjoyed. Cut out and post the
article.

➪ Write a letter to the editor of a local newspaper and tell your
story.

➪ Write a poem or little song about what took place.

➪ Encourage the person receiving care to call a friend or family
member and tell them about the enjoyable activity.

➪ Tell "tall tales" about the activity and how it went; exaggeration
can be a great source of fun and laughter.

Create your own ways to record the good times. You will be glad
you did.

Summary

Use the Checklist of Leisure Favorites as a basis for planning activities
that are favorites. Try to include activities from all of the P.I.E.S.S.
(physical, intellectual, emotional, social, and spiritual aspects of life)
in order to meet the needs of the whole person and provide a variety
of activities. Set an enjoyable activity plan for each day (or each visit).
Be flexible and ready to change plans according to changes in health
and mood and weather, as well as unexpected events. Keep the plan
simple and suited to the individual. The *process* of the activity is what

counts more than the end-products you may produce. Make the most of every phase—before, during, and after—and you'll not only have more to do together, but more to talk about and more memories to enjoy. Keep some records of the good times to keep your memories alive both now and over the years to come.

CHAPTER NINE

Parting Thoughts

Leisure is a powerful tool in safeguarding and restoring our health and wellness. This book, so far, has addressed leisure in the caregiving *relationship*. In this chapter, I want to turn my focus in a slightly different direction, and examine the importance of leisure experiences for caregivers outside of their caregiving roles. In addition, you will find the following:

☆ How caregiver support groups can provide leisure-related help
☆ How to ask for and find help
☆ A few closing thoughts about leisure for everyone

Leisure for the Caregiver

No doubt caregivers would agree with researchers who report that caregiving considerably changes the lives of those who give care, including their leisure and recreation. The U.S. Select Committee on Aging, in 1988, noted the impact of caregiving on leisure lifestyle in these words: "Caregivers tend to double up on their responsibilities and to cut back on their leisure time to fulfill all of their caregiver tasks." When life's demands require that we leave something out, leisure too often becomes that "something."

It is too bad that caregivers readily leave out leisure in their lives, because leisure plays a vital role, not only in our enjoyment of life but also in how we manage adversity that comes our way. A 1988 study of caregivers' free time by therapeutic recreation educator Janiece Sneegas, for example, found that leisure provided opportunities for caregivers to escape from their tasks and reduce tension. Sneegas also suggested that leisure activities provided a way for caregivers to cope with the burdens of their role. Also, in a 1993 study, Edward H. Thompson and his associates in the department of sociology and anthropology at Holy Cross College in Worcester, Massachusetts, assessed six types of social support in relation to caregivers' burdens and found that social interaction for fun and recreation appeared to be the most important type of social support for diminishing the caregiving burden. They further suggested that family caregivers should engage in regular, pleasant activities with friends and other family members to ease their caregiving burdens.

And yet little attention has been paid to the role of recreation and leisure as a coping strategy for caregivers. Perhaps researchers as well as caregivers pay little attention to leisure because they are uncomfortable with the idea of taking time for the caregiver when the person being cared for is not able to fully join in. Therapeutic recreation educator Leandra Bedini and activities director C. W. Bilbro have found that many caregivers feel selfish and guilty if they care for their own needs. In their 1990 study of caregivers' stress, human development and aging specialist Leonard I. Pearlin and associates at the University of California, San Francisco, urged caregivers to understand how important it is to take care of themselves in order to provide quality and appropriate care.

Taking time for self-refreshment must be seen as necessary for effective service. We cannot help others unless we have sufficient energy for the necessary tasks. In his 1988 book *Super Joy*, Paul Pearsall explains that "joy is as contagious as stress and depression," and that "our own joy is healing and helpful to others," because it energizes us to help and share with others.

If you are someone who feels guilty about taking time for yourself or having fun before all your work is done, your challenge is to change the way you think about your leisure. Perhaps you feel it is wrong to enjoy yourself while others around you, particularly the person in your care, are sick and in need. There may be a long list of reasons you give yourself for not socializing with friends or taking time for yourself, but you can change the way you think about your leisure if you want to. In 1986 Shad Helmstetter published a book called *What to Say When You*

Talk to Yourself, in which he explains the importance of using self-talk to change your thinking and behavior. His system can be useful in getting rid of the "guilties" that often come with leisure when there is still work to be done. It will take time and practice to change your thinking, but you can do it. You can practice talking to yourself like this:

✓ "I can enjoy myself and still be a good caregiver."
✓ "I deserve to have fun."
✓ "When I take care of myself I am able to take care of others better."
✓ "When I am joyful, I have joy to share with others."

Find your own words, but speak positively to yourself to change the way you think. When you think of the benefits that will come to both you and the other person by taking time for leisure, you are more likely to overcome the guilt in your mind.

Also, give yourself leisure breaks even though all your work is not finished. When was the last time all your work was finished? I mean *all* your work? Never, of course. And it never will be. Does that mean you are never allowed to take time for leisure? Certainly not. That would be absurd. Just five or ten minutes here or there will be helpful to you. A visit with a friend can give you important social support when you need it. Or, just being alone and quiet for five minutes can help you collect your thoughts and calm your nerves. A ten-minute walk in the fresh air will do you more good than a candy bar, because it will activate all your systems and give you ongoing benefits.

Walking is a handy and useful way to exercise. It can be done any-time, indoors or outdoors, requires only good shoes and no special uni-form or equipment, and it can be done alone or with others. For those who are especially motivated by the presence of other people, it is a great activity to do with a friend. Walking results in fewer injuries than other forms of exercise, while benefiting the entire body. Short, rapid walks are effective for many people to reduce anxiety, tension, and blood pressure. Walking is highly recommended for caregivers as a convenient way to exercise and manage stress.

Here are a few more ideas, which I call Leisure Lifters, for lighten-ing your days in small ways. Give yourself permission for these simple pleasures.

Leisure Lifters for Lighter Living

1. Get up in time to enjoy the sunrise; note the light, color, breeze, temperature, your own feelings of awakening.
2. Take time for a long, hot shower. Relax and enjoy the water on your body and the warmth through and through.
3. Eat your food as though for the first time. Notice and enjoy the flavors, colors, textures, crunches. Savor every bite. Eat slowly and chew each mouthful more than usual.
4. After a meal, sit and visit with family members or just sit by yourself to enjoy the moments without hopping up quickly to care for dishes or other tasks.
5. Listen to the entire song or commentary before turning off a radio or TV.
6. Make up your own words to a favorite tune and sing the words as they come to you; it's okay to be silly or sentimental.
7. Go soak your feet in comfortably hot water. Enjoy the warmth throughout your whole body. Don't move until the water is beginning to get cool.
8. Watch a sunset go *all the way* down. Note the afterglow and nature's beauty.
9. Write your own poem or draw a picture and hang it in a favorite spot.
10. Find a pretty stone while you walk. Pick it up and notice its color, surface, shape, weight, cracks; feel it between your thumb and forefinger.
11. Take time for a nap.
12. Sit outside in the night air and be at peace.
13. Give yourself a massage. Rub hand or body lotion gently into your pores wherever you have tense muscles or an ache. Take time to be good to yourself.
14. Try a new hairdo or just another way of combing your hair; see if anyone notices the change.
15. Buy yourself flowers, arrange them joyfully, and place them where you will see them often. Enjoy the colors and fragrances.
16. Step outside in the night air to look at the moon and the stars.
17. When you shop for groceries, spend a few moments in the

produce section to enjoy the colors, arrangements, and fragrances of the fruits and vegetables.

18. Warm your clothing in a dryer before dressing; relish the warmth.
19. Take a long, soaking bubble bath; dim the lights; light a candle; enjoy.
20. Warm your towels to use after a bath or shower. Ahhh!
21. Treat yourself to a hot, soothing drink of your favorite kind.
22. Listen to music and read favorite poetry, scripture, or books.
23. Talk to yourself on paper in your own private journal.
24. Now that you have the idea, add to this list and keep on practicing!

Support Groups and Leisure Education

A friend of mine cares for his brother who is living with AIDS. He and his family joined a support group to manage their own feelings and learn strategies to make their brother's life as comfortable and meaningful as possible. My friend claims the support sessions helped everyone cope and express their feelings. Yet, there came a time when they expressed all their feelings and needed something more. Leisure can provide that "something more" in two ways: it can easily fit into support groups for caregivers as (1) a topic of discussion and (2) enjoyable activity to do together.

Leisure content in the discussions of support group meetings is a vital part of nurturing leisure wellness in the caregiving process. In support groups, caregivers can not only learn how to use leisure activities to benefit their care receivers but also explore the importance of leisure in their own lives. In her 1992 book *Taking Care of Me: How Caregivers Can Effectively Deal with Stress*, Katherine L. Karr suggests that support groups are often successful because of the help members provide for each other. Because of the intimate information caregivers share in support groups, they form close bonds with each other that also help them cope better. Participating in leisure activities conveys a similar bonding effect. It can be useful, therefore, for support group members to participate together in leisure activities from time to time to help lighten each other's moods and strengthen bonds among one another.

Support group leaders are in an excellent position to help groups of caregivers address the importance of leisure in their own lives and in the caregiving process. Leisure awareness can be developed by discussing the importance of leisure, what it is, and how it can enhance life in many ways. Social and leisure skill development are best accomplished by participating in activities and learning how to do the tasks required for participation. When we know how to do activities, we are more likely to schedule them into our days and continue doing them. But sometimes we are not sure where to find the people or places to do things we enjoy. That's where leisure resource awareness comes in. By finding out what is available in our area and how to take advantage of the opportunities that match our time, resources, and lifestyles, we can learn how to go about the business of finding our own fun. These are the bits of information often missing among caregivers (and people in general) which limit their participation in a variety of leisure experiences. But if leisure information and learning opportunities are made more available, people are more likely to participate. Caregiver support groups seem to be an ideal arrangement for this kind of help.

It seems that support group members are well equipped to help each other overcome the barriers they encounter in their leisure, since they have firsthand experience with their own lack of leisure. Support group members could discuss a wide range of leisure topics such as:

⇨ Barbara Ann Kipfer's book of *14,000 Things to Be Happy About* (discussed in Chapter 2)
⇨ how to stay tuned to the daily things that bring happiness
⇨ how to plan something interesting into every day
⇨ leisure-time tips that have worked for individual members
⇨ barriers to leisure time—and how to overcome them
⇨ how to find time for yourself
⇨ finding nontraditional leisure experiences in every day
⇨ how to enjoy yourself without feeling guilty
⇨ where to learn how to do specific activities
⇨ who to contact for help with leisure activities
⇨ where to call to find out what's going on in the community
⇨ how to find free things to do for fun

The following Eighty-Eight Free Fun Things to Do will get you started. This list could be an interesting discussion topic at a support group meeting. But it can be very useful just for you. Notice how many of the suggestions fall into the "nontraditional leisure activity" category. Each of us will find some great ideas on this list and other ideas that we think should be left out. Each of us makes unique choices. Have some fun reading and discussing the list and adding to it. Do some of your favorites!

Eighty-Eight Free Fun Things to Do

Taste free samples at the grocery store

Draw a floor plan of your dream house

Kiss someone you love

Try on outfits at a clothing store

Read cards at a card shop

Read a book or two

Invite friends for a Monopoly game

Figure out how something works

Give and/or receive a back rub

Draw pictures

Color or paint something

Blow bubbles

Write a poem

Ride a bike

Visit someone

Learn to play the harmonica

Walk in the rain

Look at the moon through a telescope

Make a list of personal goals

Go to a jewelry store and try on rings

Meditate

Rearrange your closet

Browse through a bookstore

Plan a picnic

Take a hot bath

Dance in front of a mirror

Test drive cars

Visit a pet store

Organize drawers, tools, shelves

Play cards

Walk in the woods

Ask someone to give you a foot rub

Learn a magic trick

Sing

Write a song

Reminisce

Hug someone special

Read old magazines

Listen to the radio

Visit a flower shop

Star gaze

Catch fire flies, let them go

Have a garage sale

Tell stories

Order free catalogs

Look at old photos

Swim

Write letters to friends

Do some bird watching

Take a walk

Wash your car

Make cookies

Converse with someone you don't know

Look through a catalog, make a wish list

Visit the library

Plant seeds (indoors or outdoors)

Wash your pet

Take a tour of a local company

Try to teach a pet a new trick

Walk through a field

Build a fort in the woods (or snow)

Take a new route home

Make snow angels

Sit in on a class at the university

Plan and set up an experiment

Learn Origami

Make a craft item

Have a lip-sync contest

Plan a vacation

Walk, talk, sit in the park

Look up something in the encyclopedia

People watch in a mall

Have a paper airplane contest

Sit in on public court trials

Listen to music

Go around the block

Set up a lemonade stand

Plant a garden

Read a magazine

Throw away clutter

Daydream

Whistle

Press flowers or leaves in a book

Tell jokes

Pray

Watch the clouds go by

Go to a free concert

Really smell some roses

Finding Leisure Contacts

Although some support group leaders may acknowledge the importance of leisure to the caregiver, they may not be comfortable with the idea of including the leisure topic in group discussions. They may not feel well informed in this area or they may not know just how to go about the task. Leisure and recreation professionals can be of help. By contacting nearby health-care facilities, such as hospitals and nursing homes, group leaders or members can locate therapeutic recreation specialists who might be willing to participate in group meetings and assist in the leisure information process. Therapeutic recreation specialists, sometimes called recreation therapists, are professionally prepared to help persons with illness or disability meet their leisure needs. Their understanding of caregiving situations has prepared them to be of help to caregivers as well as to care receivers.

Other community recreation staff may also be of help. Community park and recreation personnel will gladly share information about local activities and events available for groups or for individual participation. Staff members at local agencies such as a YMCA or community education office may also be happy to tell support group members about their ongoing programs, fees, and special events. Most communities also have special interest groups such as garden clubs, bird watchers, hiking clubs, volleyball leagues, bowling leagues, poetry groups, and study and discussion groups. The Chamber of Commerce may be the best place to identify such special interest groups and their leaders, who can be asked to speak at a support group meeting and give members their leisure-related help and ideas.

Asking for Help

Because the tasks of caregiving are often overwhelming, it is easy to feel you are alone in all that you have to accomplish. Yet, there are a wide range of services and people available to help in many ways to make your caregiving situation more workable. Other family members, friends, and neighbors are a good place to start. Sometimes people ask what they can do to be of help, or they might say, "If there is ever anything I can do, be sure to let me know." Rather than dismissing those words as simply courteous comments, pay attention to who said that, and think about how they *really could* help out, even in little ways. "Take them up" on the offer. They may be both pleased and surprised to know there is something they can do to help.

Usually people are better able to respond to a *specific* request for help rather than just being asked to help out. You might ask them to stop in for an hour's visit and to read the newspaper to the person receiving care while you step out for a walk in the park to give yourself some exercise and quiet time. Or, perhaps a neighbor is not comfortable being alone with the other person, but will be happy to play a table game at the bedside of the care receiver while you complete other tasks. You might ask a relative who lives miles away to write frequent letters, send a poem now and then, or send updated photos of family members from time to time. A specific request will give a willing helper something definite to do, and you will feel their support as well. It is a matter of following up on their offer to help that is key to helping yourself. You don't have to do everything yourself. Don't be shy. Ask for *specific* help.

If you are looking for more general services to support your caregiving efforts, there are many other places to start:

✓ The yellow pages of your telephone book may have an information and referral "hot line" for health-care services. Call and tell them your situation, and they can lead you to other related services.
✓ Your doctor or nurse can refer you to local resources of help.
✓ The senior citizens center in your community has information about their own programs and activities as well as other services in the community.
✓ Churches, temples, and synagogues often have members organized to serve the special needs of people in their local communities.
✓ You might place a phone call to a long-term care facility, adult day care service, respite care service, or a home health-care provider to find out what kinds of services they provide and see if they can be of help in your particular situation. Even if you aren't sure about what kind of help you need, tell them your story. They will be able to let you know whether they are able to serve you, or will be able to connect you to someone else who can. If you are looking for leisure-related help when you call these agencies, ask if there is a therapeutic recreation specialist on staff, and ask him or her for the leisure help or information you need.

Leisure for Everyone

Leisure moments are important throughout our lives, when we are young, middle-aged, and old, whether we are well or ill, healthy or dying. Children have the natural spirit of play. They don't think about what their bodies, minds, or spirits need; they naturally play and, through their activities, meet those needs. Often the responsibilities of adulthood, though, bring a joyless existence of caring for ourselves and others without giving time to leisure wellness. But leisure is a significant element of health and happiness throughout our lives, not only during childhood or during times of good health. All human beings need some freedom from necessity to enjoy the kind of small pleasures featured in the following poem that was written by someone very wise, though unnamed. It was passed along to me by a friend.

Life's Tiny Delights

Most of us miss out on life's big prizes.
The Pulitzer. The Nobel. Oscars. Tonys. Emmys.
But we are all eligible for
life's small pleasures:
a handful of wild flowers,
lunch with a friend,
a kiss behind the ear,
a full moon,
an empty parking space, a crackling fire,
a golden sunset, hot soup, quiet prayer.
Don't fret about missing life's grand awards.
Enjoy its tiny delights. There are plenty for all of us!

Anonymous

Although this book has been about leisure in the caregiving process, I want to emphasize how vital it is to blend leisure into life, long before a person needs care. For everyone, leisure experiences can be something to look forward to and something to make every day worth getting up for. "Enjoying life" does not mean throwing care to the wind, being irresponsible or lazy. Rather, we can balance our responsibilities with meaningful activities that brighten and lighten life. There is a very old song that rings out this good advice: "Enjoy yourself, it's later than you think; enjoy yourself, while you're still in the pink. The years go by as quickly as a wink. Enjoy yourself, enjoy yourself, it's later than you think!"

If we are wise, we won't wait until illness, disability, pain, or impending death turn our thoughts to the importance of life's moments. We can take steps *now* to prevent regrets so we and those we love don't end up saying things like, "Too bad we didn't do such and such while he was alive" or "I wish we had done such and such while we could." Let's not put off leisure adventures whether they are simple or sophisticated. Plan and dream about them, strategize to make them happen and then enjoy the memories. When illness or disability complicates life, work with that, too, and manage to achieve even small leisure goals. On our deathbeds we won't be saying things like, "I wish I had worked another job" or "Too bad I didn't clean the house more often." Rather, if we have regrets they will sound more like: "I wish I had spent more time with my family" or "Too bad we didn't take time to have fun" or "I wish I had said I love you." *Now* is the time to listen to your heart and find your way toward leisure dreams and goals. Seize the day. Enjoy daily delights and make memories. *Make all the moments count.*

Resources

Abilitations
  One Sportime Way
  Atlanta, GA 30340
  (800) 850-8602
  Free catalog of adapted equipment for physical and mental activities available.

ABLE DATA
  National Rehabilitation Information Center
  4407 Eighth Street, N.E.
  Washington, DC 20017
  (202) 635-6090
  (202) 635-5884 (TTP)
  This is a computerized national data base for rehabilitation products.

Access to Recreation
  2509 East Thousand Oaks Blvd., Suite 430
  Thousand Oaks, CA 91362
  (800) 634-4351
  Free catalog shows a variety of adapted devices available to serve special recreation needs.

Access to Travel: A Guide to Accessibility of Airport Terminals
  U.S. General Services Administration
  Washington, DC 20405

adaptAbility
P.O. Box 515
Colchester, CT 06415-0515
(800) 266-8856
Free catalog of adapted devices for recreation and a wide range of activities
of daily living.

Alexander Graham Bell Association for the Deaf
3417 Volta Place, N.W.
Washington, DC 20007

Alzheimer's Disease and Related Disorders Association
P.O. Box 5675
Chicago, IL 60685
(800) 621-0379

American Alliance for Health, Physical Education, Recreation, and Dance
1900 Association Drive
Reston, VA 22091
(703) 476-3400

American Cancer Society, National Headquarters
1599 Clifton Road NE
Atlanta, GA 30329-4251
(800) 227-2345

American Council of the Blind, Inc.
1010 Vermont Avenue, N.W., Suite 111
Washington, DC 20005
(800) 424-8666 or (202) 393-3666
Information available about support groups for persons who are blind and
visually impaired.

American Diabetes Association, National Service Center
P.O. Box 25757
1600 Duke Street
Alexandria, VA 22313
(800) 232-3472 or (703) 549-1500

American Foundation for the Blind, Inc.
15 West 16th Street
New York, NY 10011
(800) 232-5463
They will be able to help you find general information about blindness and how to find services for persons who are blind and visually impaired.

American Parkinson's Disease Association
(800) 223-APDA

American Therapeutic Recreation Association
P.O. Box 1521
Hattiesburg, MS 39404-5215
They can provide information about recreation-related publications and can help you find a therapeutic recreation specialist in your area.

Appliances for the Physically Challenged
(800) 235-7054
Free catalog will inform you of adapted devices for various recreation needs.

Artists with Handicaps: Resources for Artists with Disabilities, Inc.
60 East 8th St., #289
New York, NY 10003
(212) 460-8510

AT&T National Special Needs Center
Parsippany, NJ 07054
(800) 233-1222
TDD (800) 833-3232

Briggs Corporation
7887 University Blvd.
P.O. Box 1698
Des Moines, IA 50306-1698
(800) 247-2343
Free catalog of adapted materials for activity and recreational therapy.

Captioned Films for the Deaf
(800) 237-6213

Cancer Information Service
(800) 4-CANCER

Communication Center
Minnesota State Services for the Blind
2200 University Avenue West #240
St. Paul, MN 55114
(612) 642-0513
They are the best contact to find out which states have radio reading
services and how you can locate them.

Enrichments 7
P.O. Box 471
Western Springs, IL 60558-0471
(800) 323-5547
Free catalog of adapted devices for recreation and activities of daily living.

Geriatric Resources, Inc.
931 South Semoran Blvd. #200
Winter Park, FL 32792
(800) 359-0390
Free catalog of sensory stimulation products designed for Alzheimer's Type
dementia and geriatric rehabilitation.

The Lupus Foundation of America, Inc., National Office
1717 Massachusetts Ave., N.W., Suite 203
Washington, DC 20036
(800) 558-0121

National Easter Seal Society
70 Eastlake St.
Chicago, IL 60601
(312) 726-6200
Publishers of *Computer Disability News* newsletter.

National Federation of the Blind
1800 Johnson Street
Baltimore, MD 21230
(301) 659-9314
They can provide information about support groups and training centers in
mobility for persons who are blind; they help to connect persons who are
blind with others who are blind for support and assistance in daily living.

National Federation of Interfaith Volunteer Caregivers, Inc.
  105 Mary's Avenue
  P.O. Box 1939
  Kingston, NY 12401
  (914) 331-1358
  They can provide information about how to find or establish an interfaith
  volunteer network in your area.

National Foundation for Hearing/Speech
  (800) 638-8255

National Multiple Sclerosis Society
  (800) 334-7812

National Organization on Disability
  (800) 248-ABLE

National Park Service
  Division of Special Programs and Populations
  Department of Interior
  18th and C Street, N.W.
  Washington, DC 20240
  (202) 343-4747
  Information available about accessible mobility on national park sites.

National Spinal Cord Injury Hotline
  (800) 962-9629

National Therapeutic Recreation Society
  2775 South Quincy Street, Suite 300
  Arlington, VA 22206-2204
  They can provide information about recreation-related publications and can
  help you find a therapeutic recreation specialist in your area.

Plasti-Dip International
  1485 West Country Road C
  St. Paul, MN 55113
  Product to dip and cover handles with rubberlike substance for easier
  gripping.

Radio Shack Catalog for People with Special Needs
    At local Radio Shack stores or from:
    300 One Tandy Center
    Fort Worth, TX 76102

Reader Enterprises, Inc.
    193 Robinson Street
    Binghamton, NY 13904
    They can send you information about a "no hands" reading stand.

Recorded Books
    (800) 638-1304

Recordings for the Blind
    (800) 221-4792

Rehabilitation International U.S.A.
    1123 Broadway, Suite 704
    New York, NY 10010
    (212) 620-4040
    They can provide publications on accessibility to cities, transportation
    systems, and hotel chains; write for "International Directory of Access
    Guide" for travelers who are disabled; send stamped business envelope.

Sunset House
    12800 Culver Blvd.
    Los Angeles, CA 90066
    Write for a catalog of gadgets for easier living plus fun items.

Therapy Dogs International, Inc.
    6 Hilltop Road
    Mendham, NJ 07945
    (201) 543-0888
    They can inform you of local groups of pet owners who have trained their
    dogs to serve persons with special needs.

United Cerebral Palsy
    (800) 872-1827

References

References Related to Caregiving Relationships and Caregivers' Stress

Abel, E. K. 1995. "Representations of caregiving by Margaret Forster, Mary Gordon, and Doris Lessing." *Research on Aging* 17 (1): 42–64.

Adler, G., M. A. Kuskowski, and J. Mortimer. 1995. "Respite use in dementia patients." *Clinical Gerontologist* 15 (3): 17–30.

Bedini, L. A., and C. W. Bilbro. 1991. "Caregivers, the hidden victims: Easing caregiver's burden through recreation and leisure services." *Annual in Therapeutic Recreation* 2: 49–54.

Braithwaite, V. 1996. "Between stressors and outcomes: Can we simplify caregiving process variables?" *Gerontologist* 36 (1): 42–53.

Cant, R. 1993. "Constraints on social activities of caregivers: A sociological perspective." *Australian Occupational Therapy Journal* 40 (3): 113–21.

Dupuis, S. L., and A. Pedlar. 1995. "Family leisure programs in institutional care settings: Buffering the stress of caregivers." *Therapeutic Recreation Journal* 29 (3): 184–205.

Hooker, K., L. D. Frazier, and D. Monahan. 1994. "Personality and coping among caregivers of spouses with dementia." *Gerontologist* 34 (3): 386–92.

Karr, K. L. 1992. *Taking Care of Me: How Caregivers Can Effectively Deal with Stress.* Buffalo, N.Y.: Prometheus Books.

Keller, M. J., and S. Hughes. 1991. "The role of leisure education with family caregivers of persons with Alzheimer's Disease and related disorders." *Annual in Therapeutic Recreation* 2: 1–7.

Kitwood, T., and K. Bredin. 1992. "Towards a theory of dementia care: Personhood and well-being." *Ageing and Society* 12: 269–87.

Lawton, M. P., E. M. Brody, and A. R. Saperstein. 1989. "A controlled study of respite service for caregivers of Alzheimer's patients." *Gerontologist* 29 (1): 8–16.

Lawton, M. P., M. Moss, and L. M. Duhamel. 1995. "The quality of daily life among elderly care receivers." *Journal of Applied Gerontology* 14 (2): 150–71.

Lieberman, M. A., and L. Fisher. 1995. "The impact of chronic illness on the health and well-being of family members." *Gerontologist* 35 (1): 94–111.

Pearlin, L. I., J. T. Mullan, S. J. Semple, and M. M. Skaff. 1990. "Caregiving and the stress process: An overview of concepts and their measures." *Gerontologist* 30 (5): 583–84.

Pearsall, P. 1988. *Super Joy*. New York: Doubleday.

Sankar, A. 1991. *Dying at Home: A Family Guide for Caregiving*. Baltimore: Johns Hopkins University Press.

Sheehan, N. W., and P. Nuttall. 1988. "Conflict, emotion, and personal strain among family caregivers." *Family Relations* 37 (1): 92–98.

Sneegas, J. 1988. "The role of leisure for caregivers of individuals with Alzheimer's Disease." Paper presented at the meeting of the annual National Recreation and Park Association Leisure Research Symposium, Indianapolis, Ind.

Stull, D. E., K. Kosloski, and K. Kercher. 1994. "Caregiver burden and generic well-being: Opposite sides of the same coin?" *Gerontologist* 34 (1): 88–94.

Thompson, E. H., A. M. Futterman, D. Gallagher-Thompson, J. M. Rose, and S. B. Lovett. 1993. "Social support and caregiving burden in family caregivers of frail elders." *Journals of Gerontology* 48 (5): S245–54.

White-Means, S. I. 1993. "Informal home care for frail black elderly." *Journal of Applied Gerontology* 12 (1): 18–33.

White-Means, S. I., and C. F. Chang. 1994. "Informal caregivers' leisure time and stress." *Journal of Family and Economic Issues* 15 (2): 117–36.

References Related to Leisure and Therapeutic Recreation

Austin, D. R. 1997. *Therapeutic Recreation Processes and Techniques*. 3d ed. Champaign, Ill.: Sagamore.

Berryman, D., A. James, and B. Trader. 1991. "The benefits of therapeutic recreation in physical medicine." In *Benefits of Therapeutic Recreation: A Consensus View*, edited by C. P. Coyle et al. Philadelphia: Temple University Press.

Cox, H. 1969. *The Feast of Fools*. Cambridge: Harvard University Press.

Coyle, C. P., W. B. Kinney, B. Riley, and J. W. Shank, eds. 1991. *Benefits of Therapeutic Recreation: A Consensus View*. Philadelphia: Temple University Press.

Godbey, G. 1994. *Leisure in Your Life: An Exploration*. 3d ed. State College, Pa.: Venture Publishing.

Kelly, J. R. 1990. *Leisure*. 2d ed. Englewood Cliffs, N.J.: Prentice-Hall.

Kraus, R., and J. Shank. 1989. *Therapeutic Recreation Service: Principles and Practices*. Dubuque, Iowa: Wm. C. Brown.

McDowell, C. F. 1983. *Leisure Wellness: Coping Strategies and Managing Stress*. Eugene, Oreg.: Sun Moon Press.

Peterson, C., and S. L. Gunn. 1985. *Therapeutic Recreation Program Design: Principles and Procedures*. 2d ed. Englewood Cliffs, N.J.: Prentice-Hall.

Riddick, C., and M. J. Keller. 1991. "The benefits of therapeutic recreation in gerontology." In *Benefits of Therapeutic Recreation: A Consensus View*, edited by C. P. Coyle et al. Philadelphia: Temple University Press.

References Related to Leisure Activities and Implementation Strategies

American Association of Retired Persons (AARP). 1989. *Reminiscence: Finding Meaning in Memories*. Social Outreach and Support Section Program of AARP.

Baer, B. 1985. "The rehabilitative influences of creative experience." *Journal of Creative Behavior* 19 (3): 202–14.

Bailey, L. M. 1984. "The use of songs in music therapy with cancer patients and their families." *Music Therapy* 4 (1): 5–17.

Birren, J. E., and D. E. Deutchman. 1991. *Guiding Autobiography Groups for Older Adults: Exploring the Fabric of Life*. Baltimore: Johns Hopkins University Press.

Carter, J. 1996. "Singing with Mom." *Reader's Digest* (August), p. 13.

———. "Songs of Innocence and Experience." *Wall Street Journal*, March 26, p. A 18.

Dancy, J., and M. L. Wynn-Dancy. 1994. "Faith of our fathers (mothers) living still: Spirituality as a force for the transmission of family values within the black community." *Activities, Adaptations, and Aging* 19 (2): 87–105.

DeSchriver, M. M., and C. C. Riddick. 1990. "Effects of watching aquariums on elders' stress." *Anthrozoos* 4 (1): 44–48.

Dorfman, R. A. 1994. *Aging into the 21st Century: The Exploration of Aspirations and Values*. New York: Brunner/Mazel.

Dossey, L. 1993. *Healing Words: The Power of Prayer and the Practice of Medicine*. San Francisco: Harper/San Francisco.

Dowling, J. R. 1995. *Keeping Busy: A Handbook of Activities for Persons with Dementia*. Baltimore: Johns Hopkins University Press.

Feil, N. 1991. *The Validation Breakthrough*. Baltimore: Health Professionals Press.

Feldman, J. S. 1993. "An alternative group approach: Using multidisciplinary expertise to support patients with prostate cancer and their families." *Journal of Psychosocial Oncology* 11 (2): 83–93.

Francis, G., and A. Baly. 1986. "Plush animals—Do they make a difference?" *Geriatric Nursing* May–June, 140–42.

Goff, K., and E. P. Torrance. 1991. "Healing qualities of imagery and creativity." *Journal of Creative Behavior* 25 (4): 296–303.

Grossman, A. H. 1996. "Acquired immunodeficiency syndrome (AIDS)." In *Therapeutic Recreation: An Introduction*. 2d ed. Edited by D. Austin and M. D. Crawford. Boston: Allyn and Bacon.

Helmstetter, S. 1986. *What to Say When You Talk to Yourself*. New York: Pocket Books.

Hunt, A. H. 1993. "Humor as a nursing intervention." *Cancer Nursing* 16 (1): 34–39.

Jackson, L. T. 1991. "Leisure activities and quality of life." *Activities, Adaptations and Aging* 15 (4): 31–36.

Khouzam, H. R., C. Smith, and B. Bassett. 1994. "Bible Therapy: A treatment of agitation in elderly patients with Alzheimer's Disease." *Clinical Gerontologist* 15 (2): 71–74.

Kipfer, B. A. 1990. *14,000 Things to Be Happy About.* New York: Workman.

Klein, A. 1989. *The Healing Power of Humor.* Los Angeles: Jeremy P. Tarcher.

Lago, D., M. Delaney, M. Miller, and C. Grill. 1989. "Companion animals, attitudes toward pets, and health outcomes among the elderly: A long-term follow-up." *Anthrozoos* 3 (1): 25–34.

Logan, A. 1985. "Soap operas and reality orientation." *Expanding Horizons in Therapeutic Recreation.* Columbia: University of Missouri.

Mayo Clinic. 1995. "Activity Therapy." *Mayo Clinic Health Letter* 13 (8): 6.

———. 1996. "Health and Spirituality." *Mayo Clinic Health Letter* 14 (11): 4–5.

McGuire, F. A., and R. K. Boyd. 1993. "The role of humor in enhancing the quality of later life." In *Activity and Aging: Staying Involved in Later Life*, edited by J. R. Kelly. Newbury Park: Sage.

McKee, P. L. 1995. "Gardening—An equal opportunity joy." *Activities, Adaptations, and Aging*, 20 (1): 71–78.

Offner, N. J. 1992. *Gentle Yoga with Naomi* (videocassette). New York: Botticelli, La Primavera, Photography: Erich Lessing / Art Resource.

Osgood, N. J. 1993. "Creative activity and the arts: Possibilities and programs." In *Activity and Aging: Staying Involved in Later Life*, edited by J. R. Kelly. Newbury Park: Sage.

Peniston, L. 1991. "The effects of a microcomputer training program on short-term memory in elderly individuals." A paper presented at the Benefits of Therapeutic Recreation in Rehabilitation Conference, Lafayette Hill, Pa.

Reynolds, B. 1996. "Prayer the medicine patients are seeking." *USA Today*, May 3, 1996, p. 1.

Shary, J. M., and S. E. Iso-Ahola. 1989. "Effects of a control-relevant intervention on nursing home residents' perceived competence and self-esteem." *Therapeutic Recreation Journal* 23 (1): 7–16.

Sherman, E. 1991. *Reminiscence and the Self in Old Age.* New York: Springer.

Sherman, J. R. 1995. *The Magic of Humor in Caregiving.* Golden Valley, Minn.: Pathway.

Siegel, B. S. 1986. *Love, Medicine, and Miracles.* New York: Harper and Row.

Siegel, J. M. 1990. "Stressful life events and use of physician services among the elderly: The moderating role of pet ownership." *Journal of Personality and Social Psychology* 58 (6): 1081–86.

Thayer, R. E. 1988. "Energy Walks." *Psychology Today* 22 (10): 12.

Tobin, S. S. 1991. *Personhood in Advanced Old Age: Implications for Practice.* New York: Springer.

Thorsheim, H. I., and B. B. Roberts. 1990. *Reminiscing Together: Ways to Help Us Keep Mentally Fit As We Grow Older.* Minneapolis: CompCare.

Weiss, C., and J. M. Thurn. 1987. "A mapping project to facilitate reminiscence in a long-term care facility." *Therapeutic Recreation Journal* 21 (2): 46–53.

Weiss, C. 1989. "Therapeutic recreation and reminiscing: The pursuit of elusive memory and the art of remembering." *Therapeutic Recreation Journal* 23 (3): 7–18.

Williams, E. M. 1994. "Reality Orientation Groups." In *Working with Older Adults: Group Process and Techniques.* 3d ed. Edited by I. Burnside and M. G. Schmidt. Boston: Jones and Bartlett.

Zgola, J. 1987. *Doing Things: A Guide to Programing Activities for Persons with Alzheimer's Disease and Related Disorders.* Baltimore: Johns Hopkins University Press.

Index

Library of Congress Cataloging-in-Publication Data
  Decker, Joanne Ardolf.
    Making the moments count : leisure activities for caregiving
  relationships / Joanne Ardolf Decker.
       p.   cm.
    Includes bibliographical references (p.   ) and index.
    ISBN 0-8018-5699-X (alk. paper). — ISBN 0-8018-5700-7
  (pbk.)
    1. Recreational therapy.   I. Title.
  RM736.7.D43 1997
  615.8'5153—dc21   97-12488
                                                         CIP

Decker, Joanne
Ardolf.

**Making the moments
count.**

DATE			